D1294698

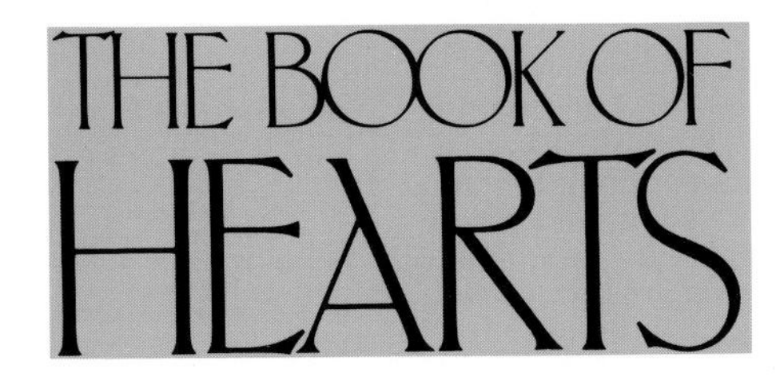

Running Press
Book Publishers
Philadelphia, Pennsylvania

Canadian representatives: General Publishing Co., Ltd.
30 Lesmill Road, Don Mills, Ontario M3B 2T6.

9 8 7 6 5 4 3 2
The digit on the right indicates the number of this printing.

Library of Congress Cataloging in Publication Data:
The Book of Hearts.
Summary: Quotations, stories, recipes, quizzes, and little-known facts about the heart.
1. Heart. 2. Heart—Anecdotes, facetiae, satire, etc. [1. Heart—Miscellanea]
QP111.4.B66 1983 612'.17 83-13957

ISBN: 0-89471-446-5 cloth

Cover design by Toby Schmidt.
Cover illustration by Lauren E. Simeone.
Illustration by Judith K.M. Barbour.
Typography: Weiss, with Plantin and Univers,
by rci, Philadelphia, Pennsylvania.
Printed in Hong Kong by Leefung Asco Ltd.

Acknowledgements

Grateful acknowledgment is made to the following for permission to reproduce materials. In the listing below, titles preceded by an asterisk are not part of the original copyrighted material.

*A Hearty Dish from India: From *Cooking of the Maharajas,* by S.R. and S.D. Holkar; © 1975 by The Viking Press. *The Walking Heart: From "Walking," by Jack Galub, *Glamour,* June 1978; copyright © 1978 by The Conde Nast Publications, Inc. Heart-Burial: Reprinted with permission from *Encyclopaedia Britannica,* 11th edition, © 1910–11 by Encyclopaedia Britannica, Inc. *Never Bet the Devil Your Heart: From *The Enlarged Devil's Dictionary,* © 1967 by Ernest J. Hopkins; reprinted by permission of Doubleday & Company. *The Unabridged Heart: Reprinted by permission from *Webster's Third New International Dictionary* © 1976 by G. & C. Merriam Co., Publishers of the Merriam-Webster Dictionaries. A Man All Heart: From *A Dictionary of British Folk-Tales,* by Katharine M. Briggs; Part A, Folk Narratives, Vol. 2; copyright © 1970 by K.M. Briggs; reprinted by permission of Indiana University Press. *Reflections on Heart Transplants: From *Biological Systems,* by Shelby D. Gerking; © 1974 by W.B. Saunders Company. *The Purest Theatre; *The Bower of Love; The Garrulous Heart: From *Mortal Lessons,* copyright © 1974, 1975, 1976 by Richard Selzer; reprinted by permission of Simon & Schuster, a Division of Gulf & Western Corporation. *Cross My Heart: copyright © 1976 by The New York Times Company; reprinted by permission. *The Nutritious Heart: Reprinted by permission from *Barbara Kraus Dictionary of Protein,* © 1975 by Harper & Row, Publishers, Inc. Pickled Venison Heart; Pickled Elk's Heart: Reprinted by permission of G.P. Putnam's Sons from *The New York Times Heritage Cook Book* by Jean Hewitt; copyright © 1972 by The New York Times. *Heartbroken: Reprinted with permission from *Stedman's Medical Dictionary,* © 1961 by The Williams & Wilkins Company, Baltimore.

This book may be ordered by mail from the publisher. Please include $1.00 postage.
But try your bookstore first.
Running Press
Book Publishers
125 South 22nd Street
Philadelphia, Pennsylvania 19103

THE BOOK OF HEARTS

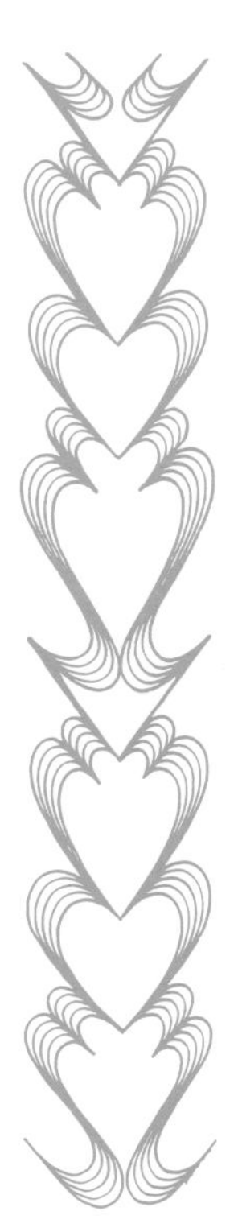

"Perhaps," muses surgeon-author Richard Selzer, "if one were to cut out a heart, a lobe of the liver, a single convolution of the brain, and paste it to a page, it would speak with more eloquence than all the words of Balzac. Such a piece would need no literary style, no mass of erudition or history, but in its very shape and feel would tell all the frailty and strength, the despair and nobility of man. What? Publish a heart? A little piece of bone? Preposterous. Still I fear that is what it may require to reveal the truth that lies hidden in the body."

In a sense, the heart of man embodies his truth, his strength, his nobility. In this book, we invite you to share some of the eloquence, whimsy, and knowledge inspired by the ten ounces of beating muscle which is the pulse of every human life. Surely *The Book of Hearts* will show you the myriad ways in which the mind expresses its fascination with the heart.

What's a Heart Like?

The diversity of things to which the heart has been compared does more than tickle the imagination: it courts it. For example:

The heart of a man has been compared to flowers; but unlike them, it does not wait for the blowing of the wind to be scattered abroad.
—*Yohida Kenko*

The heart is like an instrument whose strings steal nobler music from life's many frets.
—*Gerald Massey*

Her heart, like the lake,
was as pure and as calm,
Till love o'er it came,
like a breeze o'er the sea,
And made the heart heave
of sweet Mary machree.
—Samuel Lover

The heart of a man is like a delicate weed,
That requires to be trampled on boldly indeed.
—*Anon.*

The hearts of pretty women, like New Year's bonbons, are wrapped in enigmas.—*J. Petit-Senn*

My heart is like fire in a close vessel: I am ready to burst for want of vent. —*John Wesley*

A maiden's heart is as champagne, ever struggling upward.—*C.S. Calverley*

A woman's heart is as intricate as a ravelled skein of silk. —*Dumas Père*

The human heart is like Indian rubber: a little swells it, but a great deal will not burst it.
—*Anne Bronte*

My heart is like a singing bird
Whose nest is in a watered shoot;
My heart is like an apple-tree
Whose boughs are bent with thickset fruit;
My heart is like a rainbow shell
That paddles in a halcyon sea;
My heart is gladder than all these
Because my love is come to me.
—Christina Rossetti

The Language of the Heart

Unlearn'd, he knew no schoolman's subtle art,
No language, but the language of the heart.
—Alexander Pope

If an international gossip column reported the exchange of *hjerte* for *sziv* between a Danish lady and a Hungarian gentleman, we'd have to suppose that some kind of knot had been tied: perhaps the suturing-up after a bit of fancy surgery—perhaps the intertwining of amorous souls.

Arabic	qalb *(tr)*	*Norwegian*	hjerte
Czech	srdce	*Polish*	serce
Danish	hjerte	*Portuguese*	coracao
Dutch	hart	*Rumanian*	inima
Esperanto	koro	*Russian*	syertse *(tr)*
Finnish	sydan	*Serbo-Croatian*	srce
French	coeur	*Spanish*	corazon
German	herz	*Swahili*	moyo
Greek	kardia *(tr)*	*Swedish*	hjarta
Hebrew	lev *(tr)*	*Turkish*	kalb
Hungarian	sziv	*Yiddish*	herts *(tr)*
Indonesian	annutdjg		
Italian	cuore		

tr—transliteration

THE UNABRIDGED HEART

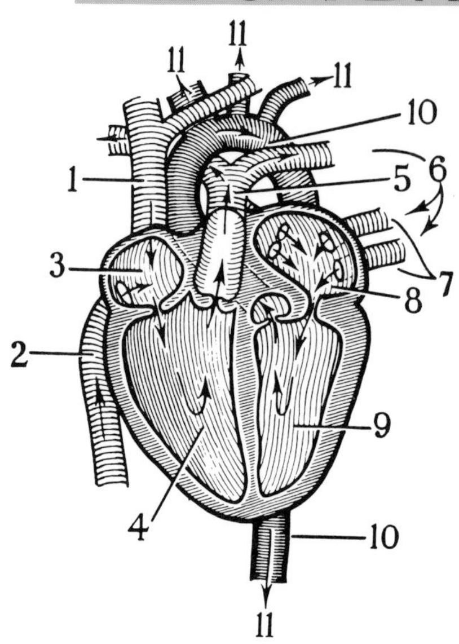

heart 1a, showing course of the blood coming from the body and entering from *1* superior vena cava and from *2* inferior vena cava; to *3* right atrium; to *4* right ventricle; to *5* pulmonary artery; to *6* lungs (not shown); to *7* pulmonary veins; to *8* left atrium; to *9* left ventricle; to *10* aorta; leaving by *11* to the head, neck, and upper extremities (not shown)

[1]**heart**\ ˈhärt, ˈhȧt, *usu* -d. + V\ *n* -s [ME *hert*, fr. OE *heorte*; akin to OHG *herza* heart, ON *hjarta*, Goth *hairto*, L *cord-*, *cor*, OIr *cride*, Gk •*kardia*, Arm *sirt*, Hitt *karts*] **1 a:** a hollow muscular organ of vertebrate animals that by its rhythmic contraction acts as a force pump maintaining the circulation of the blood, is in the human adult about five inches long and three and one half broad, of conical form, is placed obliquely in the chest with the broad end upward and to the right and the apex opposite the interval between the cartilages of the fifth and sixth ribs on the left side, is enclosed in a serous pericardium, and consists as in other mammals and in birds of four chambers divided into an upper pair of rather thin-walled auricles which receive blood from the veins and a lower pair of thick-walled ventricles into which the blood is forced and which in turn pump it into the arteries, back flow being prevented by valves, or in lower forms is less perfectly differentiated, having usu. two auricles and one ventricle in reptiles and amphibians and but a single auricle and ventricle in most fishes **b :** a structure in an invertebrate animal functionally analogous to the vertebrate heart: as **(1)** : a contractile ventricle with one to four thin-walled auricles that circulates the body fluid of most mollusks **(2)** : a contractile tube in most arthropods that receives blood from an investing pericardial sinus through openings provided with valves and circulates it forward and peripherally in the body **(3)** : any of a series of paired pulsating anterior blood vessels connecting the main dorsal and ventral blood vessels of certain annelids **c :** BREAST, BOSOM <could have hugged him to my ~—W.M. Thackeray> **d :** something resembling a heart in shape: **(1)** : a conventionalized representation of a heart (as a decorative figure or a trinket) **(2)** : a red conventionalized figure of a heart stamped on a playing card **(3)** : a heart-shaped block through which a lanyard is reeved to extend stays **(4)** : the heart-shaped part of a pound net placed at the end of the

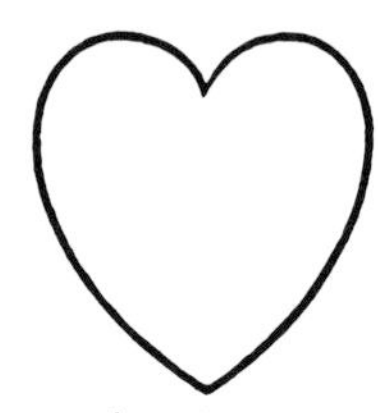

heart 1d(1)

leader to direct fish into the pot (5) : a foundry molder's heart-shaped trowel (6) **hearts** *pl but sing in constr* : **a wood sorrel** *(Oxalis montana)* **2 a :** a playing card marked with a conventionalized figure of a heart **b : hearts** *pl* : the suit comprising cards so marked **c :** an odd bridge trick won or contracted for when hearts are trumps **d : hearts** *pl but sing in constr* : a game resembling whist in which the object is to avoid taking tricks containing hearts and often other specified cards **3 a** (1) : the whole personality including intellectual as well as emotional functions or traits <come from the ~ that is gay, warm, friendly, and enthusiastic —Constance Foster> <I say what is in my ~> <deep in your own ~, you share my prejudice—Walter de la Mare> <each man knew in his ~ that it was a lie—L.B. Salomon> (2) *obs* : INTELLECT, UNDERSTANDING (3) : MEMORY, ROTE—used in the phrase *by heart* <got the whole poem by ~> <knew the town's 500 telephone numbers by ~—Peg Bracken> (4) : OPINION, ATTITUDE, POSTURE—used chiefly in the phrase *change of heart* <two aspects to the Soviet change of ~ on the Austrian treaty—T.P. Whitney> **b** (1) : the emotional or moral as distinguished from the intellectual nature : CONSCIENCE, CHARACTER, SPIRIT <has a good ~ but a weak head> <who can look into the ~ of a man> <his ~ dictated one course, his reason another> (2) : generous disposition : SENSIBILITY, COMPASSION, FEELINGS <have you no ~> <Oh, have a ~, lend me a dollar> (3) : hardness or flintiness of character or temper : unfeeling disposition—usu. used with *have* in negative construction <he loved his wife; he had not the ~ to deny her anything—Clara Morris> <hadn't the ~ . . . to refuse to come—Ellen Glasgow> (4) : TEMPERAMENT, DISPOSITION, MOOD <went home with a heavy ~> <are not inclined to regard free-trade agitation with a light ~—*Dun's Rev.*> (5) : GOODWILL, WILLINGNESS, SINCERITY, ZEAL—used chiefly in the phrase *with all my heart* <will do it for you with all my ~> **c :** LOVE, AFFECTIONS <he lost his ~ to her at once> <laid his ~ at her feet> <a free public-school system . . . was one thing that lay near his ~—A.W. Long> <his speeches won him ~s from coast to coast—William Clark> **d :** COURAGE, ARDOR, ENTHUSIASM <don't lose ~; all will turn out well> <felt some sinking of the ~> <an unsatisfactory . . . student, for my ~ was not in it—W.S. Maugham> <put ~ into me by what you say—O.W. Holmes †1935> <at the sight of reinforcements, the dispirited soldiers took ~> <lost all ~ for my silly chase—Arthur Grimble> <many a people has kept itself in ~ when its statesmen have despaired—W.B. Adams> **e** (1) : TASTE, LIKING <likes music but has no ~ for grand opera>—used chiefly in the phrase *after one's own heart* <a man after his own ~> (2) : fixed purpose or desire : ardent wish—now used chiefly in the phrase *set one's heart on* <set his ~ on getting a new car> (3) : intense concern, solicitude, or preoccupation—used chiefly in the phrase *at heart* <people who are unaware of the issue which he has at ~—J.H. Robinson> <with victory secured, there was one other thing that he had at ~> **f :** one's innermost being : one's innermost or actual character, disposition, or feelings—used chiefly in the phrases *at heart* <at ~ a sensitive high-strung man> and *heart of hearts* <assisting those who in their ~ of hearts are . . . implacably anti-American—Perry Miller> <in his ~ of hearts I do not think he ever really surrenders faith—Edward Wagenknecht> **4 :** PERSON <two young ~s had been freed . . . from the burden of guilt and suspicion—Agnes S. Turnbull>—usu. used with a qualifier <poor ~! who would relieve her wants now> <farewell, dear ~> **5 :** the central or decisive part of something : CENTER : as **a :** an inner central area or region <a system of waterways extending into the ~ of No. America> **b :** an essential part : the part that determines the real nature of something or gives significance to the other parts : the determining aspect <the discernment and understanding with which he penetrates to the ~ and essence of the problem—B.N. Cardozo> <those words of Jesus show us the ~ of Easter's meaning—W.F. Hambly> **c :** the center of activity : a vital part on which continuing activity or existence depends <Rome was the ~ and pulse of the empire—John Buchan> **d :** HEARTWOOD **e :** CORE 1h **f :** a firm part (as of a head of lettuce); *also* : the center of a celery plant **6** *chiefly Brit* : condition for bearing crops : FERTILITY—used chiefly in the phrase *in good heart* <the land has never been in better ~—S.P.B. Mais> **syn** see CENTER — **to heart** *adv* : under serious consideration : with deep concern : with hurt feelings <took it *to heart*> <Sterne . . . laid the criticism *to heart*—Virginia Woolf>—**to one's heart's content :** to the point of complete satisfaction or satiety : to the limits of one's will or pleasure <eat *to your heart's content*> <printers imported any foreign books they thought would be popular . . . and reprinted them *to their heart's content*—Margaret Nicholson>

All who know their own minds, do not know their own hearts.

–François de La Rochefoucauld

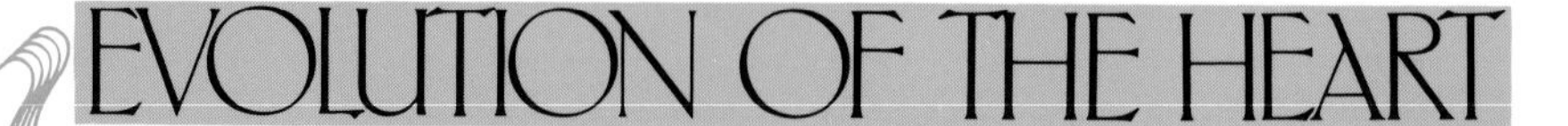

EVOLUTION OF THE HEART

The heart, ready furnished with its proper organs of motion, like a kind of internal creature, existed before the body. The first to be formed, nature willed that it should afterwards fashion, nourish, preserve, complete the entire animal, as its work and dwelling-place: and as the prince in a kingdom, in whose hands lie the chief and highest authority, rules over all, the heart is the source and foundation from which all power is derived, on which all power depends in the animal body. . . .

Thus nature, ever perfect and divine, doing nothing in vain, has neither given a heart where it was not required, nor produced it before its office had become necessary; but by the same stages in the development of every animal, passing through the forms of all, as I may say (ovum, worm, foetus), it acquires perfection in each. —William Harvey

The first heart was also the simplest. Some 450 million years ago, when life was still restricted to the vast oceans, some tiny primitive creatures had become sufficiently complex to require a circulatory system to pump oxygen through their bodies. After a long period of evolution, the first heart developed into a long, narrow vessel with a regular pulsation. As living things became more complex, the circulatory system kept pace, culminating in the most complex, efficient, and spectacularly engineered heart of all, that of the mammal.

This development can be retraced by examining the hearts of more ancient forms of life. The ancestral heart could support creatures no more than several inches long. From this first primitive heart and its successors came the two-chambered heart, still found in fish, in which blood collects in one

HEARTBEATS PER MINUTE

Blue whale	*5 to 6*
Turtle	*6 to 70*
Elephant	*22 to 50*
Fish	*40 to 80*
Human	*70 to 75*
Rabbit	*100 to 300*
Bird	*200 to 1000*
Mouse	*300 to 500*
Shrew	*500 to 1000*

chamber and is then propelled into the second, which in turn contracts and pushes the blood out into the circulatory vessels. This heart made it possible for much larger forms of life to develop in the oceans.

The two-chambered heart fulfilled the needs of most sea creatures, but species moving onto the fringes of the land required a more efficient circulatory system. Creatures of the land developed lungs, which necessitated a rearrangement of the heart. And thus evolved the three-chambered heart still found in amphibians and most reptiles. In this heart, oxygen-rich blood from the lungs is carried to one chamber; oxygen-poor blood coming from the rest of the body enters another. The third chamber draws alternately from these two chambers, pumping oxygen-rich blood to the rest of the body and sending oxygen-poor blood to the lungs to pick up a new supply.

The three-chambered heart emerged about 300 million years ago. Some 100 million years later (give or take 5 million years), the four-chambered heart of the mammals was first developed. Because birds and mammals are warm-blooded, they use up oxygen at a much more rapid rate than other creatures. To meet this pressing need for oxygen, a fourth heart chamber evolved. The existence of this fourth chamber means that oxygen-rich blood and oxygen-poor blood will never mix: each is sent to a different chamber and routed on its way, either to the lungs or the body. This much more efficient arrangement crowns the 300-million-year evolution of the heart.

A Definition, by Ambrose Bierce

In each human heart are a tiger, a pig, an ass, and a nightingale. Diversity of character is due to their unequal activity. –Ambrose Bierce

HEART, *n.* An automatic muscular bloodpump. Figuratively, this useful organ is said to be the seat of emotions and sentiments—a very pretty fancy which, however, is nothing but a survival of a once universal belief. It is now known that the sentiments and emotions reside in the stomach, being evolved from food by chemical action of the gastric fluid. The exact process by which a beefsteak becomes a feeling—tender or not, according to the age of the animal from which it was cut; the successive stages of elaboration through which a caviar sandwich is transmuted to a quaint fancy and reappears as a pungent epigram; the marvelous functional methods of converting a hard-boiled egg into religious contrition, or a creampuff into a sigh of sensibility—these things have been patiently ascertained by M. Pasteur, and by him expounded with convincing lucidity. (See, also, my monograph, *The Essential Identity of the Spiritual Affections and Certain Intestinal Gases Freed in Digestion*—4to, 687 pp.) In a scientific work entitled, I believe, *Delectatio Demonorum* (John Camden Hotton, London, 1873) this view of the sentiments receives a striking illustration; and for further light consult Professor Dam's famous treatise on *Love as a Product of Alimentary Maceration.*

HEART-A-FACTS

The human heart accounts for about 1/200th of the total body weight.

Bigger people have bigger hearts.

Sudden happiness increases the heart rate. So does sudden anger. Initially, an experience of fear lowers *the heart rate.*

In one minute, the heart pumps between 8 and 10 pints of blood through 60,000 miles of blood vessels—that's more than twice the distance around the world.

The heart rate is at its highest in the early afternoon and at its lowest in the morning.

The heart beats continuously from the fifth month before birth until death.

Each heartbeat lasts about eight-tenths of a second.

On the average, the human heart beats 72 times a minute, or about 100,000 times a day, or about 38,000,000 times a year, and about 4 billion times during an average lifetime.

In one day, the heart pumps the equivalent of 5,000 gallons of blood through the body.

THE HEART AS A SYMBOL

It would be easier to list the cultures in which the heart has *not* been used in a variety of symbolic ways than to enumerate those in which it has attained importance. Throughout recorded history, stylized portraits of the heart have symbolized certain qualities and beliefs in art and literature. Cultures widely distant in both time and place seem to have attributed very similar meanings to the heart.

Again and again, the heart is used to represent the focus, the *center* of a

CAVE HEART

Veterinary anatomy might be a relatively new field of study, but the cave art of our Paleolithic ancestors some 20,000 years ago shows that the position—and the significance—of the hearts of hunted beasts were well understood. Drawn more or less like the now traditional, symmetrical form, the hearts of the elephant and the bison, for example, are clearly depicted and accurately placed within the outline drawing of the entire animal. In these mostly detail-free pictures, the inclusion of the heart bespeaks the cavedwellers' ritualistic belief that the power to conquer an adversary begins to take shape with the ability to capture its image.

human being, the source from which all intelligence and emotions flow. The Sumerians believed the heart to be the site of human intelligence. This perception may have been at least partly based on the early realization of the heart's importance in the body, since even the oldest civilizations seem to have known far more about the functionings of the heart than those of the brain. So, just as the physical heart maintained the body, it was thought that the spiritual heart was the source of man's other qualities.

The Egyptian Book of the Dead *devotes six chapters to the heart, the only visceral organ to be retained when a body was mummified. It was crucial that the heart accompany the deceased to the netherworld since his fate would be decided when Osiris weighed the heart in his judgment hall.*
The Egyptians believed that blood vessels carried and filtered not only blood but also human waste. It was thus possible for such wastes to be carried to the heart and damage it.

What began as essentially religious beliefs were gradually diffused and adapted in each different culture. In the East, many came to identify the heart as a symbol of wisdom and spiritual realization:

The heart of a wise man should resemble a mirror, which reflects every object without being sullied by any. —*Confucius*

Heart failure, wounds of the heart, and fainting caused by heart malfunction are all described accurately in the Old Testament. In addition, the relation of a healthy heart to longevity, the manner in which the heart functions and its centrality in the body functions are also mentioned. These descriptions indicate a high level of knowledge about the physical workings of the heart among Near Eastern cultures as early as 2,500 years ago.

Ancient Hindus believed that by concentrating his meditation upon the heart, the ascetic (or yogi) was able to probe not only his own mind but those of others. The philosopher Shankara says that this concentration should be "in the form of a light the size of the thumb situated in the cavity of the heart."

In the Old Testament, the heart is understood to be the center and source of each human being, the point from which thought, emotions, and will all emanate, and the organ which focuses the function of conscience. It is from the heart that all a person's actions originate. Understanding, imagination, determination, and memory all have their origin in the heart. Virtue and vice, humility and pride, good and evil thoughts and deeds, all come from the heart.

Man looketh at the outward appearance, but the Lord looketh on the heart.

—I Samuel 16:17

The heart of a man changeth his countenance, whether it be for good or evil.

—Ecclesiasticus 10:7

The Heart of Dionysus

Dionysus is remembered today as the Greek god of wine and ecstasy. In fact, the beliefs centering on Dionysus were considerably more complex. He was also worshipped as a certain proof of the resurrection and survival of the soul after death. Central to this belief were tales explaining Dionysus' death and remarkable resurrection. And in many of these tales, the heart of Dionysus had a central place.

Although tales describing Dionysus' death differ, all agree on the manner of his death: he was torn to pieces, which were either widely scattered or consumed by the supernatural creatures that had murdered him. In some versions, Dionysus' mother, the goddess Semele, succeeded in gathering all the pieces of his body together, and reanimated them. In the versions in which his body is consumed by his enemies, only his heart is preserved from his foes' appetites. Then Zeus, most powerful of all the gods, either swallows the heart and then begets Dionysus again upon Semele, or he causes the heart to be reduced to a powder, mixed in a potion and given to Semele. And from the potion she again conceives and gives birth to Dionysus.

Belief in the immortality of the soul was an important tenet of the Dionysian faith. And the heart, as symbol of the core of each human personality, representative of the soul, understandably became the focus of the tales concerning this belief.

In the West, the heart became an emblem of lovers, identified as the source of either amorous or religious love.

"The Greek physiology did not divide the Self by the polarity of 'brain' and 'heart' as popular fantasies distinguish these organs of rational thinking and sympathetic feelings. In the Greek concept of the Self the brain was not valued as highly as by primitive head-hunters and modern neurologists. . . . The intellectual capacity of man was thought to be located in the heart. The internals, and especially the heart, were considered as the undivided incarnation of man's intellectual and emotional qualities. This may be the expression of a most primitive concept of the Self. It is noteworthy that the Egyptian deities are represented with animal heads and human bodies, while in the Greek fantasies the personifications of instinctual drives appear as human above the diaphragm, as animal below it."

—Theodore Thass-Thienemann

The heart and the eyes, explains the troubadour poet Aimeric de Peguilhan, are the organs of love: "True Love, I assure you, has not, and cannot have of himself, force or power, or any authority either small or great, unless the eyes and the heart give it to him. . . . For the eyes are the dragoman of the heart, and the eyes seek out what it pleases the heart to retain; and when they are well accorded all three, and firmly of one mind, then True Love is born from that which the eyes make pleasing to the heart. . . . And so, let all true lovers know that Love is a true affection which is born of the heart and of the eyes, without doubt, that the eyes make it flower and the heart causes it to bear fruit—Love, the fruit of the true seed."

Heart's Magic

Many ancient cultures considered the heart to be the seat of power that controlled other areas of the body. It was believed to be equidistant from the brain and the genitals, and this position enabled it to balance both. "One will grant the heart a modicum of history," writes Dr. Richard Selzer. "Ancient man slew his enemy, then fell upon the corpse to cut out his heart, which he ate with gusto, for it was well understood that to devour the slain enemy's heart was to take upon oneself the strength, valor and skill of the vanquished."

Among the Iroquois, it was considered a great honor for a warrior to be awarded the heart of a brave prisoner taken in battle. By eating the heart, the victor believed that he would assume some of his enemy's courage. Sir James Frazer's *The Golden Bough* records many such instances of primitive belief in the homeopathic magic of a fleshy diet—better known as a hearty meal.

"In Morocco lethargic patients are given ants to swallow, and to eat lion's flesh will make a coward brave; but people abstain from eating the hearts of fowls, lest thereby they should be rendered timid."

"When Basutos [an African tribe] of the mountains have killed a very brave foe, they immediately cut out his heart and eat it, because this is supposed to give them his courage and strength in battle. When Sir Charles M'Carthy was killed by the Ashantees in 1824, it is said that his heart was devoured by the chiefs of the Ashantee army, who hoped by this means to imbibe his courage."—Sir George Frazer

"The Bushmen will not give their children a jackal's heart to eat, lest it should make them timid like the jackal; but they give them a leopard's heart to eat to make them brave like the leopard. When a Wagogo man of East Africa kills a lion, he eats the heart in order to become brave like a lion; but he thinks that to eat the heart of a hen would make him timid."

"The Ainu believe that the heart of the water-ousel is exceedingly wise, and that in speech the bird is most eloquent. Therefore whenever he is killed, he should be at once torn open and his heart wrenched out and swallowed before it has time to grow cold or suffer damage of any kind. If a man swallows it thus, he will become very fluent and wise, and will be able to argue down all his adversaries."

"In Norse legend, Ingiald, son of King Aunund, was timid in his youth, but after eating the heart of a wolf he became very bold; Hialto gained strength and courage by eating the heart of a bear and drinking its blood."

"A North American Indian thought that brandy must be a decoction of hearts and tongues, 'because,' said he, 'after drinking it I fear nothing, and I talk wonderfully.' "

"The Indians of Guayaquil, in Ecuador, used to sacrifice human blood and the hearts of men when they sowed their fields."

Food of the Gods

When the Aztecs spoke of the "food of the gods," they were referring to the human heart —and not in any symbolic way. Their gods were hungry gods, demanding a steady diet of hearts in return for keeping the universe in order.

The Aztecs' domination of central Mexico lasted only a little more than a hundred years, ending when they were overthrown by Cortes and his conquistadores in the 16th century. But in that short span of time, the Aztecs may have sacrificed hundreds of thousands of people to their gods.

Every year, some fifteen thousand prisoners (most of them captured during the Aztecs' many wars and raids) were led up to the temples atop the great stone pyramids. There they were spreadeagled on a sacrificial stone and killed by the single stroke of an obsidian knife which tore the hearts from their bodies. The hearts were then ritually offered to the gods and cast into a brazier to be burned.

HOW COYOTE STOLE GOD'S HEART

California's Yuman Indians tell of how their god died, poisoned by an evil and envious being. The people mourned bitterly. Now that they had lost their god, death had finally come among them.

Coyote wanted the heart of the god because he believed it would make him strong. He tried every trick he could think of to steal the heart away, but the people always beat him back. During the god's cremation ceremony, however, just as the body was about to be consumed by the flames, Coyote made a great leap onto the funeral pyre, snatched the heart, and ran away with it.

One tribe of California Indians, the Juaneno, had a mourning ritual in which this folk tale figured. Since the "heart" of a dead person was understood to be the soul, when anyone died a figure acting as the ano *(Coyote) would cut a piece of flesh from the dead person's shoulder and eat it. In this ritual, the flesh represented the heart, and by eating it the soul was released. It could then leave the body and ascend to the sky, where it became a star.*

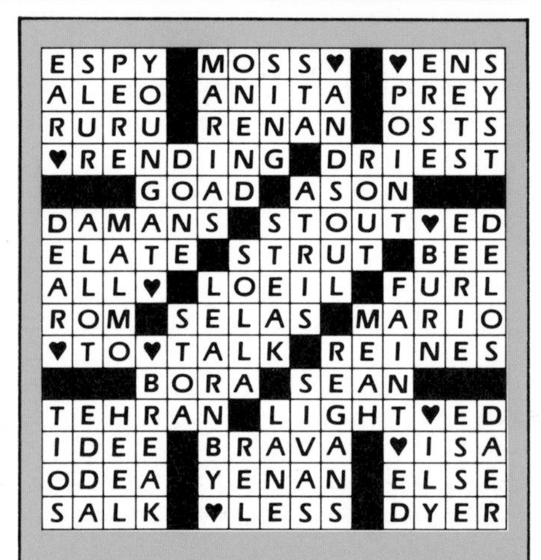

Answer to crossword puzzle on page 95.

THE NUTRITIOUS HEART

Type of Heart	Measure or Quantity	Protein (grams)	Calories
Beef:			
Lean, raw	*1 lb.*	*77.6*	*490*
Lean, braised	*4 oz.*	*35.5*	*213*
Lean, braised, chopped or diced	*1 cup (5.1 oz.)*	*45.4*	*273*
Lean with visible fat, raw	*1 lb.*	*69.9*	*1148*
Lean with visible fat, braised	*4 oz.*	*29.3*	*422*
Calf, raw	*1 lb.*	*68.0*	*562*
Calf, braised	*4 oz.*	*31.5*	*236*
Chicken, raw	*1 lb.*	*84.4*	*608*
Chicken, simmered	*1 heart (5 grams)*	*1.3*	*9*
Chicken, simmered, chopped, or diced	*1 cup (5.1 oz.)*	*36.7*	*251*
Hog, raw	*1 lb.*	*76.2*	*513*
Hog, braised	*4 oz.*	*34.9*	*221*
Lamb, raw	*1 lb.*	*76.2*	*735*
Lamb, braised	*4 oz.*	*33.5*	*295*
Turkey, raw	*1 lb.*	*73.5*	*776*
Turkey, simmered	*4 oz.*	*25.6*	*245*
Turkey, simmered, chopped, or diced	*1 cup (5.1 oz.)*	*32.8*	*313*

Pickled Venison Heart

1 venison heart
4 quarts water
2 teaspoons salt
¼ teaspoon poppy seeds
¼ teaspoon celery seeds
¼ teaspoon black peppercorns
1 clove garlic, crushed
1 teaspoon thyme
½ teaspoon marjoram
1 bay leaf
1 bottle chianti
Horseradish
Jewish pumpernickel

1. Cut a three-quarter-inch slice off the top of the heart. Mix two quarts of the water with one teaspoon of the salt. Soak heart two hours in mixture. Clean out all the blood. Drain.

2. Place heart in a saucepan with remaining water and add the poppy seeds, celery seeds, peppercorns, garlic, thyme, marjoram, bay leaf and remaining salt. Bring to a boil and simmer, covered, until heart is very tender. Cool and let stand in refrigerator two days.

3. Pour off top of broth, leaving about two cups in the bottom with most of the seasonings. Pour in the wine so that it covers the heart and let set in the refrigerator at least a week.

4. Slice very thinly and serve with horseradish and Jewish pumpernickel.

Yield: *One dozen to two dozen servings.*

Pickled Elk's Heart

1 elk's heart, well cleaned
2 teaspoons whole cloves
1 bay leaf
4 cups cider vinegar
1 tablespoon salt
1 onion, sliced
½ teaspoon dry mustard

1. Place the elk's heart in a deep saucepan and cover with water. Bring to a boil, cover and simmer until tender, about three hours.

2. Measure two cups of the cooking liquid and add remaining ingredients to it. Bring to a boil and cool.

3. Drain the heart and place in the cooled vinegar mixture so that heart is submerged. Soak ten days to two weeks in a cool place. Slice thinly.

Yield: *One dozen servings.*

A Hearty Dish from India

- *1 lb. heart (approximately 4–5 lamb hearts or 1 veal heart)*
- *1 cup unpeeled garlic cloves*
- *1 tablespoon powdered cumin*
- *2 tablespoons ground sweet fennel,* or *2 tablespoons whole fennel, coarsely ground in blender*
- *⅓ cup clarified butter*
- *2 cups onion, cut in half from top to root, and across the grain into thin, even slices*
- *½ teaspoon salt*
- *½ teaspoon powdered cardamom*

1. Two hours before serving, wash the hearts under cold running water; trim off any fatty covering and tubes, but leave the heart whole. Cover with cold water in a small saucepan and bring to rolling boil. Discard this water; rinse the hearts thoroughly and repeat this procedure once again.

2. Drop the garlic and cumin into the blender and add ½ cup water. Blend and scrape to a paste. Coat the blanched and rinsed hearts in this paste and leave thus, unrefrigerated, until they are to be cooked (minimum 1 hour).

3. After they have marinated, rinse the hearts thoroughly. Cover with cold water in a small saucepan; add the fennel and again bring to a boil. Then reduce the heat and simmer uncovered for 10 minutes. Discard the water; rinse the hearts and slice as thinly as possible with a sharp knife.

4. Preheat oven to warm (200° F.). Heat the butter in a medium-sized casserole and fry the onions until brown but not crisp. Stir in the slices of heart, salt, and cardamom. Cover and leave in a warm oven for 15–20 minutes.

Yield: *2 to 3 servings.*

Absence makes the heart grow fonder. –Thomas Haynes Bayly

Absinthe makes the heart grow fonder. –Addison Mizner

Absence makes the heart go yonder. –Charles Lee

THE MAN WITHOUT A HEART

A Popular Tale from the Norse

There were once seven brothers, who had neither father nor mother. They lived together in one house and had to do all the household work themselves, for they had no sisters. Growing lonely, they wanted companions, and one said: "Let us set out, and each of us get a wife."

This idea pleased the other brothers, and they made themselves ready for traveling, all except the youngest, who preferred to remain at home and keep house. His six brothers, promising to bring him a wife, then set out and went forth merrily in the wide world. They soon came into a wild forest, where they found a small house, with an old man standing at the door. On seeing the brothers pass by, he called to them: "Where are you bound that you pass my door so merrily?"

"We are going to fetch each of us a young bride," answered they. "We are all brothers, but have left one at home, for whom we are also to bring a bride."

"I wish you then success in your undertaking," replied the old man. "However, I too have need of a wife, and so bring me one also."

Thinking the old man spoke only in jest, the brothers made no answer, but continued on their way. They soon arrived in a city, where they found seven young and handsome sisters. Each of the brothers chose one, and took the seventh with them for their youngest brother.

When they again arrived in the forest, there stood the old man at his door, awaiting their coming. "Well," he called, "have you brought me a wife as I desired you?"

"No," answered they, "we have brought brides only for ourselves, and one for our youngest brother."

"You must keep to your promise," said the old man, "and leave her to me."

This the brothers refused to do. The old man then took a little white staff from a shelf over the door. When he touched the six brothers and their brides, they were all turned into gray stones. These, together with the staff, he laid on the shelf above the door, but kept the seventh young bride for himself.

The young woman had now to attend to all that was to be done in the house. But how was she to release her six poor enchanted sisters and their betrothed husbands? She was incessantly crying in the old man's ear: "Thou art old, and mayest die suddenly, and what am I then to do ? I shall be left alone here in this great forest."

The old man at length said: "Thou hast no cause to be uneasy. I cannot die, for I have no heart in my breast."

The young woman now appeared contented and asked him, that as his heart was not in his breast, where he kept it.

"My child," answered the old man, "be not so inquisitive. Thou canst not know everything." But she never ceased her importunities, until he at last said, somewhat peevishly, "To make thee easy, I tell thee that my heart lies in the coverlet."

Now it was the old man's custom to go into the woods every morning and not return till evening, when his young housekeeper prepared supper for him. On his return one evening, finding his coverlet adorned with beautiful flowers, he asked the young woman the meaning of it. "Oh, father," answered she, "I sit here the whole day alone, and so thought I would do something for the delight of thy heart, which lies in the coverlet!"

"My child," laughed the old man, "that was only a joke of mine. My heart is not in the coverlet, but in a very different place."

She then began again to weep and lamented, "Thou hast then a heart in thy breast, and canst die! What am I then to do, and how shall I recover my friends when thou art dead?" "I tell thee," answered the old man, "that I cannot die, and have positively no heart in my breast." She then implored him so long to inform her where he kept his heart, that he at length said: "It is in the room-door."

The following day, she decorated the room-door with flowers from top to bottom. When the old man came home in the evening and inquired the cause, she answered: "Oh, father, I sit here the whole day, and wished therefore to give some delight to thy heart." But the old man answered as before: "My heart is not in the room-door: it is in a very different place."

As on the previous day, she began to weep and implore, and said: "Thou hast then a heart and canst die; thou wilt only deceive me."

The old man answered, "As thou wilt positively know where my heart is, I will tell thee. Very far from here, in a wholly solitary place, is a large church secured by thick iron doors. Around it runs a wide, deep moat. Within the church there flies a bird, and in that bird is my heart. So long as that bird lives, I also live. Of itself it will not die, and no one can catch it. Hence I cannot die. But even if I should die, which is not possible, there lie the 12 gray stones over the door, together with a little white staff. Thou hast only to strike the stones with that stick, and all thy friends—thy sisters and their betrothed—will again be living."

In the meantime, the youngest brother had waited at home. As his brothers did not return, he therefore set out in quest of them. After traveling for some days, he arrived at the house of the old man. He was not at home, but the young woman received him. He related to her how his six brothers had all left home to get themselves wives, but that some mischance must have befallen them. The young woman then instantly knew him for her bridegroom, and informed him what had become of his brothers and their brides. She gave him food to eat, and when he had recruited his strength, he said: "Tell me, my dear, how can I release my brothers?" She then related to him all about the old man whose heart was not in his breast but in a far distant church, of which she gave him every particular, according to the old man's narrative.

"I will try to get hold of the bird," said the young man. "The way is long and the church well secured, but by God's help I may succeed."

"Do so," said the young woman, "for as long as the bird lives, thy brothers cannot be released." Accordingly, she gave him a whole basketful of provisions, and after a tender farewell, he resumed his journey.

He had proceeded a considerable way when, feeling hungry, he sat down, placed his basket before him, took forth some bread and meat, and said: "Let come now every one that desires to eat with me!" At the instant came a huge red ox and said, "I would gladly eat with thee."

"Very well," said the young man, "and thou shalt partake with me."

They then began to eat, and when they were satisfied, the red ox said, "If at any time thou requirest my aid, thou hast only to utter the wish, and I will come and help thee." He then disappeared among the trees.

When the young man had proceeded a considerable way farther, he was again hungry, so he sat down, opened his basket, and said as before: "Let those come that desire to eat with me!"

In a moment a large wild boar came from the thicket and said: "I would gladly eat with thee." When they had eaten, the boar said: "If ever thou needest my aid, only utter the wish, and I will help thee." He then disappeared in the forest, and the young man pursued his journey.

On the third day, when about to eat, he said again, "Come all that desire to eat with me!" At the instant a rattling was heard among the trees and a large griffon descended by the side of the traveler, saying, "If thou didst say that all who desired to eat with thee might come, I would gladly eat with thee."

"With all my heart," answered the bridegroom; " 'tis far more pleasant to eat in company than alone."

When their hunger was satisfied, the griffon said: "If ever thou art in difficulty, only call me and I will aid thee." He then disappeared in the air, and the young man went his way.

After traveling a while longer he perceived the church at a distance. But now there was the moat in his way. "The red ox could help," thought he, "if he were to drink the water. Oh, that he were here!" Hardly had he expressed the wish when the red ox was there, laid himself on his knees and drank until there was a dry path through the water.

The young man now stood before the church. Its iron doors were so strong that he could not force one open, and the walls many feet thick, without an opening in any part. "Oh," he cried, "if the wild boar were here!" In an instant it came rushing up, and ran with such force that in one moment a large hole was broken through the wall, and the young man entered the church. Here he saw the bird flying about. "I cannot catch it myself," thought he, "but if the griffon were here!" Scarcely had he uttered the thought, when the griffon seized the little bird, gave it into the young man's hand and flew away. Overjoyed, he placed his prize in the basket and set forth back to the house in the forest.

When he informed his bride that he had the bird in his basket, she was overjoyed: "Now thou shalt creep under the bed with the bird, so that the old man may know nothing of the matter." And just as he had crept under the bed, the old man returned home, complaining that he felt ill.

The young woman began to weep and said: "Ah, now wilt thou die, that I can well see!"

"Ah, my child," answered the old man, "be still only; I cannot die; it will soon pass." The bridegroom under the bed now gave the bird a little pinch, and the old man grew quite pale and sat down. And when the young man squeezed it yet harder, the old man fell to the earth in a swoon. The bride then cried out: "Squeeze it quite to death." The young man did so, and the old man lay dead on the floor.

The young woman then drew her bridegroom from under the bed, and took the stones and the little white staff from the shelf over the door. She struck every stone with the staff, and in one instant, there stood before her all her sisters and the brothers. "Now," said she, "the old man is dead, and there is nothing to fear. We will set out for home, and celebrate our marriage and be happy."

And so they did, and lived many years happily in harmony together.

HEART ROOTS

English-language words related historically to the word *heart* come to us from three main linguistic branches. These all have a common origin in the hypothetical Indo-European mother tongue of many of the world's languages. Thus the postulated Indo-European form *kerd,* meaning heart, branched out into several directions, giving rise to the proto-heart word in the Germanic, Hellenic and Italic tongues.

From the Germanic stem *herton* we derive our modern term and all its obvious relatives. From the Hellenic *kardia* (heart, stomach, spirit, ego) we get scientific terms such as cardiac, pericardium, and a host of other anatomical variations. From the Italic branch, via the Latin *cor* (heart), we derive such words as cordial, courage, discord, and record, all having some concept of heart at their root. Our verb *record,* for example, comes from the Latin *recordari,* (to remember); the derivation implies that the act of remembering was originally considered a function of the heart—we do learn things "by heart"—and this is consistent with the frequent use in many older languages of a single word for both the mental and emotional functions.

Other offshoots of the Indo-European *kerd* made comparatively few contributions to the English vocabulary. One isolated example is the word *machree,* which comes via the Celtic branch from the Old Irish *cride* (heart). This form evolved into the later Irish *mo chroidhe* (my heart) and finally gave rise to *machree,* a term of endearment now used in the sense of "my dear."

Heorte, Herte, Heart

The monumental *Oxford English Dictionary* covers the origins, meanings, and uses of the vocabulary of the English language. Along with definitions, the *OED* records the earliest known context in which each word entered our language as it evolved from Anglo-Saxon to modern English over the course of roughly nine centuries.

For *heart,* the *OED* supplies 54 definitions (taking up 13 columns of type), giving the first known use, as well as later uses, of each meaning. The first recorded instance of the word heart—*heorte,* that is—in Old English dates back to 825 A.D.; the word is used to denote the center of the body's vital functions. The earliest documented use of *heorte* as an organ of the body is from the year 1000 A.D.

During the Middle English period (the 12th through 15th centuries), radical linguistic changes were caused by political, social, religious, and literary influences. In this period, the word appears variously as *he(o)rt, herte,* and *hart,* and its expanded scope of meanings becomes evident. The development of printing in the 16th century was the most important factor directing the stabilization of our ancestral language into modern English. From this time on, the form *heart* is encountered widely and in most of the senses common today.

Dr. Johnson Defines Heart

"When a butcher tells you his heart bleeds for his country, he has, in fact, no uneasy feeling."
—Samuel Johnson

Dr. Johnson's *Dictionary of the English Language* (1755), the first authoritative, comprehensive work of its kind in English, gives 21 meanings or usages for the term *heart.* To this list the pioneering lexicographer adds a few dozen popular compound heart terms.

HEART. (1) The muscle which, by its contraction and dilation, propels the blood through the course of circulation, and is therefore considered as the source of vital motion. (2) It is supposed in popular language to be the seat sometimes of courage, sometimes of affection, sometimes of honesty, or baseness. (3) The chief part; the vital part; the vigorous or efficacious part. (4) The inner part of any thing. (5) Person, character; used with respect to courage or kindness. (6) Courage, spirit. (7) Seat of love. (8) Affection; inclination. (9) Memory. (10) Good-will; ardour or zeal. To take to heart any thing, is to be zealous or solicitous or ardent about it. (11) Passion; anxiety; concern. (12) Secret thoughts; recesses of the mind. (13) Disposition of mind. (14) The heart is considered as the seat of tenderness; a hard heart therefore is cruelty. (15) To find in the heart; to be not wholly averse. (16) Secret meaning; hidden intention. (17) Conscience; sense of good or ill. (18) Strength; power; vigour; efficacy. (19) Utmost degree. (20) Life. For my heart seems sometimes to signify, if life was at stake; and sometimes for tenderness. (21) It is much used in composition for mind, or affection.

HEART-ACHE. Sorrow; pang; anguish of mind.

HEART-BREAK. Overpowering sorrow.

HEART-BREAKER. A cant name for a woman's curls, supposed to break the heart of all her lovers.

HEART-BREAKING. Overpowering with sorrow; overpowering grief.

HEART-BURNED. Having the heart inflamed.

HEART-BURNING. 1. Pain at the stomach, commonly from an acrid humour. Discontent; secret enmity.

HEART-DEAR. Sincerely beloved.

HEART-EASE. Quiet; tranquility.

HEARTS-EASE. A plant.

HEART-FELT. Felt in the conscience.

HEART-PEAS. A plant with round seeds in form of peas, of black colour, having the figure of a heart of a white colour upon each.

HEART-QUELLING. Conquering the affection.

HEART-RENDING. Killing with anguish.

HEART-ROBBING. Depriving of thought.

HEART-SICK. 1. Pained in mind. 2. Mortally ill; hurt in the heart.

HEART-SORE. That which pains the mind.

HEART-STRING. The tendons or nerves supposed to brace and sustain the heart.

HEART-STRUCK. 1. Driven to the heart; infixed for ever in the mind. 2. Shocked with fear or dismay.

HEART-SWELLING. Rankling in the mind.

HEART-WHOLE. 1. With the affections yet unfixed. 2. With the vitals yet unimpaired.

HEART-WOUNDING. Filling with grief.

HEARTED. It is only used in composition, as, hard-hearted.

To HEARTEN. 1. To encourage; to animate; to stir up. 2. To meliorate or renovate with manure.

HEART-WOUNDED. Filled with passion of love or grief.

PHRASES OF THE HEART

after one's heart
bless your heart
a change of heart
chicken-hearted
down-hearted
from the bottom of the heart
hale and hearty
half-hearted
heart-felt
a heart of gold
heart-rending
heart-sick
heart-to-heart talk
heart-whole
heart of stone
hearts of oak
heavy at heart
in one's heart of hearts
near to one's heart
next to the heart
out of heart
sick at heart
soft-hearted
to be at the heart of
to be deep in the heart of
to be down in the heart
to be of good heart
to be the heart and soul of
to break one's heart
to do one's heart good
to eat one's heart out
to find in one's heart to
to give heart to
to give one's heart
to have a hard heart
to have a heart
to have a soft heart
to have a soft place in the heart for
to have at heart
to have one's heart in one's mouth
to have one's heart in the right place
to have the heart to
to keep heart
to learn by heart
to lose heart
to lose one's heart
to make one's heart leap
to one's heart's content
to pluck out the heart of the mystery
to pluck up heart
to put in good heart
to put one's heart into
to search the heart
to set one's heart at rest
to set one's heart on
to take heart
to take heart of grace
to take to heart
to touch the heart of
to warm the cockles of the heart
to wear one's heart on one's sleeve
to win someone's heart
with all one's heart
with half a heart
with heart and hand
with one's whole heart
whole-hearted

SOME OFFBEAT HEARTS

Heartburn: *a bad cigar.*
Heart's ease: *a twenty-shilling piece.*
Hearts: *amphetamines.*
Heart bag: *a heart-shaped tobacco pouch.*
Hearts of oak: *penniless; broke.*
Heartbreaker: *a lovelock, a loose ringlet worn over the shoulders, or curl over the temples. Also, a flirt.*

TRAEH?

In their spare time, secretaries at the G. & C. Merriam Company, publishers of Merriam-Webster Reference Books, index entries backwards *from their* Third New International Unabridged Dictionary. *To whom might this backward file, as they call it, be of use? Well, some people just can't resist reading a new detective novel from the end forward; and others—an insatiable cardiophile, for example—may simply enjoy perusing an authoritative list of English terms and phrases ending with the word heart. Notice the (reverse) alphabetical sequence in the list which G. & C. Merriam kindly furnished us:*

heart
septemic heart
deadheart
red heart
cloistered heart
firm red heart
boxed heart
round-heart
irritable heart
purpleheart
white heart
change of heart
line of heart
bleeding heart
floating heart
lymph heart
blackheart
bullock heart
demerara greenheart
broken heart
lion heart
brown heart
mechanical heart
artificial heart
branchial heart
greenheart
tobacco heart
pseudo-heart
heart-to-heart
tiger heart
athlete's heart
bullock's heart
lion's heart
mother's heart
soldier's heart
smoker's heart
greatheart
sweetheart
left heart
right heart
faintheart
hollow heart
oxheart
pulmonary heart

A MANY-HEARTED GARDEN

Stands the lilac bush tall-growing with heart-shaped leaves of rich green. —Walt Whitman

Heartweed, or *Polygonum persicaria,* is named for the heart-shaped markings on its leaves.

Wild ginger, *Asarum canadense,* or Canada snakeroot, is also known as heart snakeroot.

Spotted medic, *Medicago maculata,* is also known as heart trefoil because of its obcordate leaflets and the somewhat heart-shaped purple or flesh-colored spot on each leaflet. It is also called heart clover or heart leaf.

Self-heal, *Brunella vulgaris,* is also called heart-of-the-earth.

Heart pea or heartseed is a general name of plants of the genus *Cardiospermum* (the English name is a translation of the Greek), but more especially of *C. halicacabum,* a beautiful vine well known among horticulturists. In the United States it is called the balloon vine, a name derived from its large, triangular, inflated fruit. The genus takes its name from the white, heart-shaped scar which marks the attachment of the seed.

The heart-leaved tway-blade is a small orchid found in the British Isles and North America.

The heart-leaved cucumber tree, a magnolia found in the southern U.S., takes its name from the cordiform shape of its leaves. It has been observed that people desire this tree as much for its symmetrical form as for the beauty of its flowers and its luxuriant foliage.

The salad known as heart of palm is made from the buds of the cabbage palmetto.

The heartnut, *Juglans sieboldiana cordiformis,* is also known as the Japanese walnut.

Sweet cherries are sometimes called heart cherries because of their shape.

When the wood in a tree begins to die and the walls of its cells harden, it is called heartwood. Heartwood is of no use to a tree except as a support. Because of its hardness and dryness, it is frequently used for industrial purposes. Heart shake is a defect in timber that occurs when one or more splits cross the center of a tree.

The heart urchin is a heart-shaped sea urchin. The name describes any spatangoid. The heart urchin is also sometimes known as mermaid's head.

The heart shell is a bivalve mollusk of the family *Isocardiidae* or *Glossidae.* The name *Isocardia cor* comes from the heart-shaped contour of the valves when viewed from the front.

The heart seine is a net with a heart-shaped enclosure or pound which can be used to catch fish however the tide may run. The enclosure itself is called a heart net.

The Indians at Hudson's Bay called the magpie the heart bird because of the shape of the large black area on its breast.

THE HEART AS RELIGIOUS SYMBOL

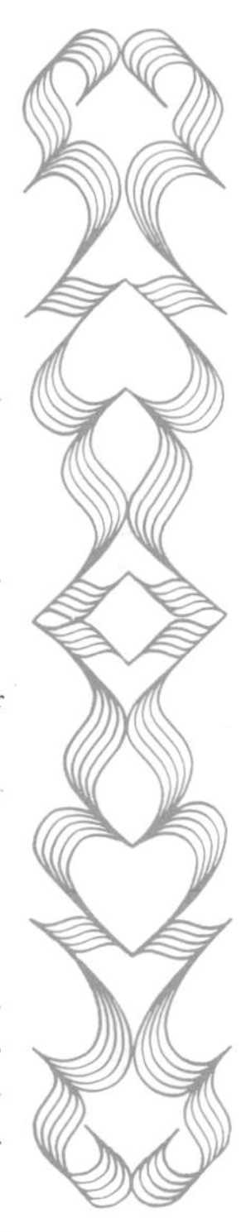

The belief in the primacy of the heart was carried through into the New Testament, and was adopted as a tenet of the Christian church as it was first formed. Indeed, the heart is referred to repeatedly by Jesus—the "pure in heart" are those who will see God; people having "honest and good" hearts are the soil in which the seeds of righteousness will grow. Hidden within the heart are those qualities which will reveal the person to be either pure or impure. And only God can read the truth engraved in each heart.

But what comes out of the mouth proceeds from the heart, and this defiles a man. For out of the heart come evil thoughts, murder, adultery, fornication, theft, false witness, slander.
—Matthew 15:18

In his *Lives of the Saints* (1623), Edward Kinesman writes, "St. Anthony of Padua, preaching a funeral sermon over a rich man of very penurious habits, took for his text *Where your treasure is, there will your heart be also.* St. Anthony said, 'This is obviously true, inasmuch as the heart of the deceased would not be found in his dead body, but in his moneybags.' Search being made, sure enough there was no heart in the dead body, but in one of the largest of the moneybags there was the dead man's heart, as fresh as if it had only that moment been removed from the carcass."

The heart is also a familiar motif in religious art. In Christianity it is often a symbol of love, piety, and charity. Abstract renderings of the heart have been adapted as ornaments to church architecture, but the heart's main use is as a symbol in painting and sculpture. A flaming heart is meant to communicate religious fervor, and when held in the hands of a saint, it symbolizes human love of God.

The image of the Sacred Heart of Jesus, represented as a flaming heart, probably dates back to the early Middle Ages. It has an important place in the sacred art of the Jesuits, in which Jesus is sometimes shown parting his garments to reveal the flaming heart in the middle of his breast. The flaming heart surrounded by thorns is also used to represent the Sacred Heart of Jesus, while the flaming heart pierced by seven knives represents the sorrows of the Blessed Virgin.

When the flaming heart is pierced by an arrow, it symbolizes repentance of sin and devotion to faith under great trials. Both the flaming heart and a heart pierced by an arrow are attributes of St. Augustine. The heart is also associated with St. Theresa and St. Bernadine. When the heart is seen with a cross, it refers to the story in which Christ appeared in a vision to St. Katherine of Siena and replaced her heart with his own.

Aristotle believed that the heart was the source of man's thoughts and emotions, and controlled the rest of the body. This was accomplished through a network of slender threads that linked it to all the other muscles—and was probably the source of the expression "tugging at one's heart strings."

ST. VALENTINE'S DAY

St. Valentine's Day can be traced back to several different kinds of celebrations all held on or about the 14th of February. Gradually, they were absorbed into a unique holiday that borrowed from each festival.

The oldest of these is the Roman feast of the Lupercalia, held as far back as the third century B.C. in honor of the god Lupercus, protector of shepherds and their flocks. When Christianity became the prevailing religion, many popular pagan holidays were transformed into religious holidays, and pagan gods were replaced by Christian saints. Thus the Lupercalia became St. Valentine's Day, in remembrance of several Christians of that name martyred by the Romans.

So the date of the holiday comes from the Romans, and the name from the early Christians, but what about its close identification with lovers? This seems to have begun with legends crediting the early martyrs with earthly as well as spiritual love. Over the years, they became not only examples of religious fortitude but patrons of lovers as well.

During the Middle Ages, many folk customs became associated with St. Valentine's Day. There was, for instance, the very old belief that birds chose their mates on February 14th. From this came the practice in which all unmarried men and women of a community drew the names of their "valentines" out of a box. This did not mean that a man and a woman would become sweethearts, but it did oblige the man to wear his valentine's name on his sleeve and serve as her protector during the next year.

From the selection of valentines, it was only a short step to the exchange of presents. And it stands to reason that the heart—symbol for thousands of years of love, fidelity, and honesty—should be used in these gifts as the symbol most appropriate to the day.

Love, Theft, and the Heart

. . . She has seen clearly the treachery of him who pretended he was a faithful lover while he was a false and treacherous thief. This thief has traduced my lady, who was ill prepared for any evil, and to whom it never occurred that he would steal her heart away. Those who love truly do not steal hearts away; there are, however, some men, by whom these former are called thieves, who themselves go about deceitfully making love, but in whom there is no real knowledge of the matter. The lover takes his lady's heart, of course, but he does not run away with it; rather does he treasure it against those thieves who, in the guise of honourable men, would steal it from them. But those are deceitful and treacherous thieves who vie with one another in stealing hearts for which they care nothing. The true lover, wherever he may go, holds the heart dear and brings it back again.

–Chretien de Troyes

THE ALLEGORY OF THE BODY AND THE HEART

An Arthurian Vignette, by Chretien de Troyes

"My lord Yvain is so distressed to leave his lady that his heart remains behind. The King may take his body off, but he cannot lead his heart away. She who stays behind clings so tightly to his heart that the King has not the power to take it away with him. When the body is left without the heart it cannot possibly live on. For such a marvel was never seen as the body alive without the heart. Yet

this marvel now came about: for he kept his body without the heart, which was wont to be enclosed in it, but which would not follow the body now. The heart has a good abiding-place, while the body, hoping for a safe return to its heart, in strange fashion takes a new heart of hope, which is so often deceitful and treacherous.''

A MAN ALL HEART: A Merry Old Tale

A northern man there was which went to seek him a service. So it happened that he came to a lord's place, which lord then had war with another lord. This lord then asked this northern man if that he durst fight. ''Yea, by God's bones,'' quod that northern man, ''that I dare, for I is all heart.'' Whereupon the lord retained him into his service.

So after, it happened that his lord should go fight with his enemies, with whom also went this northern man—which shortly was smitten in the heel with an arrow, wherefore he incontinently fell down almost dead. Wherefore one of his fellows said: ''Art thou he that art all heart, and for so little a stroke in the heel now art almost dead?''

To whom he answered and said: ''By God's soul I is heart—head, legs, body, heels, and all—therefore ought not one to fear when he is stricken in the heart?''

A Renaissance Heart

The heart in itself is not the beginning of life; but it is a vessel formed of thick muscle, vivified and nourished by the artery and vein as are the other muscles.

Of the heart: This moves of itself and does not stop unless for ever.
—Leonardo da Vinci

Leonardo da Vinci, artist, architect, inventor, perhaps the greatest of all the great men of the Renaissance, was also a tireless student of the human body. A superb, self-trained anatomist, he made many original contributions to the field. While every part of the body held his fascination and received his close attention, he returned again and again to the study of the heart.

He compared the heart and its importance to the earth.

The lake of blood that lies about the heart is the ocean. Its breathing is by the increase and decrease of the blood in its pulses, and even so in the earth is the ebb and flow of the sea. And the vital heat of the world is fire which is spread throughout the world. . . .

The 14th century alchemist and physician Paracelsus had believed that the heart heated the rest of the body. On this matter, it was Leonardo's belief that the temperature of the blood was kept warm by

the movement of the heart, and this manifests itself because in proportion as the heart moves more swiftly the heat increases more, as is shown by the pulse of those suffering from fever which is moved by the beating of the heart.

He was wrong in this but he would have needed medical equipment much more sophisticated than any in existence at that time to discover the more subtle causes of body temperature.

Leonardo also noted that the heart acted independently of any human action. And he noted:

> *The heart . . . moves three thousand five hundred and forty times in each hour in the process of opening and shutting. And it is this frequency of movement which warms the thick muscles of the heart, and this heat warms the blood that continually beats within it. It heats it more in the left ventricle, where the walls are very thick, than in the right ventricle, with the thin wall. And this heat makes the blood grow thinner and turns it to vapor and changes it into air, and would change it to elemental fire, if it were not that the lung renders help at this crisis with the coolness of its air.*

THE HEART IN THE CUP OF GOLD

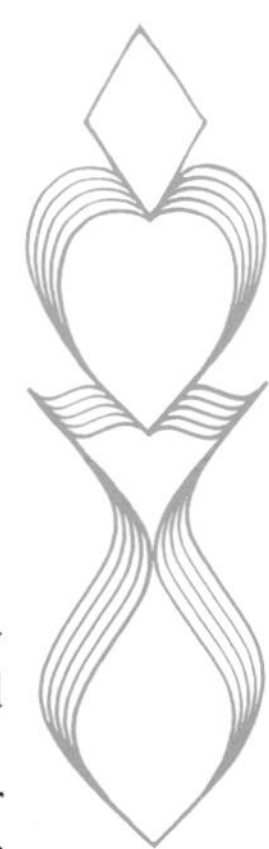

from THE DECAMERON *by Boccaccio*
retold by Richard E. Nicholls

Tancred, the ruler of Salerno, was wise and humane, and his memory would be honored today, were it not that his hands became soiled by blood (including that of the person he most loved in the world).

He had but one child, a daughter named Ghismonda, and never did father love child more. Indeed, his affection for his daughter was so great that he would become unsettled whenever she was out of his sight. For this reason, he found any number of objections to suitors for his daughter's hand. At length he was forced to consent to a marriage between his daughter and the son of the Duke of Capua. But his son-in-law died quite suddenly and his widowed daughter returned to her father's palace.

Ghismonda was a beautiful woman, quietly disposed, and possessed of a fine mind. Perceiving that her father's affection was so great that he would never allow her to remarry, but being nonetheless desirous of male companionship, she decided that if she could she would secure herself a lover.

Her father's court saw a constant coming and going of brave gentlemen (and others of inferior quality), and she carefully observed their carriage and demeanor. One especially impressed her—a servant named Guiscardo, not noble by descent, but possessing the innate nobility of the virtuous. None other pleased her as Guiscardo did, and secretly she fell in love.

Though poor, Guiscardo was not insensitive and soon realized the meaning of the way she gazed upon him. He, in turn, fell deeply in love with her. She desired nothing more than to be alone with him, yet dared not take anyone into her heart's confidence. So to satisfy her desire (which grew ever more intense), she wrote a letter, explaining how their tryst could be brought about, and placed it in the joint of a hollow cane. Then, in a jesting manner she threw it to Guiscardo, saying, "Let your man make use of this, in place of a bellows, when he comes to make a fire in your chamber." Guiscardo took up the cane, discovered the message hidden in it, and fell to following all those instructions contained in the letter, so that he might meet with the mistress of his heart.

In a corner of the palace, it being sited on a hill, there was a cave, hollowed out of the earth and illuminated by a small opening. A secret stairway, sealed by a strong door, led from the lady's apartment down to the cave. The cave and the door were largely forgotten, and the overgrown entrance to the cave could be reached only by someone lowered on a rope. Guiscardo provided himself with a rope ladder, wrapped himself in a leather cloak to avoid being scratched by brambles, and at night lowered himself into the cave.

The next morning, on the excuse of being very tired, Ghismonda sent away her serving women and retired to her chambers. Then with hurried step she went down into the cave and found there her amorous friend. Ascending into the lady's chambers, they spent the better part of the day in the ways known to lovers. When at last they had to part, Guiscardo went down and Ghismonda made fast the door behind him. Guiscardo used his rope ladder to climb out, being careful to cover the entrance of the cave behind him.

Fortune, envious of the pleasures and secrets of lovers, soon brought grief to them.

Tancred was in the habit of visiting his adored daughter's chambers. Going in one day and finding her absent, he became drowsy. Lying down at the foot of his daughter's bed, he drew the curtains about him (so he was entirely disguised) and fell asleep. Soon after, Ghismonda came in, locking the door behind her, and threw open the door to the cave. She and Guiscardo did as they were wont to do, taking their delight, and their voices awakened the prince.

Confounded by what he heard and overcome with fierce grief, he formulated a plan for revenge, and for this end remained silent, fighting back the desire to make outcry. The two lovers remained in each others' arms a long time. When they arose and took tender farewell of each other, Guiscardo went back down into the cave, and Ghismonda unlocked the door and went back to her ladies. Though old and none too spry, Tancred climbed out a window and lowered himself down into the garden.

That night, by his orders, Guiscardo was arrested as he climbed out of the cave wrapped in his leather coat. The prince had Guiscardo brought before him, and upbraided him for the base way in which he had repaid the prince's friendship. Guiscardo hung his head, and would only answer: "Love is more powerful than you or I."

Guiscardo was confined. The next day Tancred went to his daughter and confronted her with his discovery. "Ghismonda," he cried, "I always believed you the most virtuous of women, and could never have been shaken by even the worst reports. You cannot imagine the heartbreak I feel at your corrupt behavior. Yet if you must indulge in such weaknesses, could you not at least have chosen a man of your own station? With him I know how to proceed, but know not how to treat you. While nature, in its guise of paternal love, pleads pardon for you, yet justice demands punishment. To determine my course, say what you can for yourself." Having spoken, he hung down his head and wept.

Ghismonda, though faint with grief at the certain fate of her lover, yet showed marvelous strength (as love sometimes gives). Determined not to outlive Guiscardo, she faced her father unafraid. Thus she spoke:

"Father, I will not deny what has been said. True, I love Guiscardo. As long as I live—and I know that will not be long—I will love him. And if love survives death, I will love him then. I was drawn to this love not by any weakness, but by your refusal to allow me to remarry. You should remember that your daughter is of flesh and blood, and possesses the normal needs of youth. I should not have to resist the desires of the flesh: and as I yielded to them, I fell in love.

"I did not choose Guiscardo on a fancy, as many women select their lovers, but was drawn by his character. And I believe that he who lives virtuously is the truest sort of noble, no matter what his parentage. If you would compare your nobles to Guiscardo without prejudice, you would have to agree that he possesses all those qualities that make a man truly noble, and for which he should be praised.

"I care not what you do to me. I will not beg forgiveness for only having followed the dictates of my heart. Indeed, I tell you now that if you do not do to me what you do to Guiscardo, I shall inflict it on myself with my own hands. Go then and weep, and if you would kill him, favor me by killing me with the same stroke."

Tancred left his daughter, much amazed by her resolute behavior. But he did not believe she could be so determined as to kill herself, and decided to cool her ardor by punishing her in other ways.

That night he had Guiscardo strangled, and the lover's heart was cut out and carried to Tancred. Next day he had it placed in a gold cup, and sent it to his daughter. She, meanwhile, fearing the worst, had secretly obtained poisonous herbs and roots, and distilled from them a fatal draught. When she was presented with the cup and saw the heart within, she knew that Guiscardo was dead and that she must follow.

She spoke tenderly to the heart, letting her tears fall upon it. Again and again she kissed her lover's heart. Her women, astonished at Ghismonda's tears, were so moved by the sight that they too broke into lamentations. Then Ghismonda took up the poison, poured it into the golden cup, and fearlessly drank the draught. Having drained the cup, she lay down upon her bed, arranged her body modestly, and silently waited for death to release her.

Tancred, being sent for, realized what his daughter had done. Then did he weep so uncontrollably that he could not utter a word. His daughter asked simply that she and Guiscardo be buried together. Then, knowing that her end had come, she clutched her lover's heart to her and said simply, "God be with you, and let me go."

Tancred, overcome with the results of his wrath, lived for but a short time, and that time filled with grief. As Ghismonda had wished, the lovers were buried together, and all Salerno mourned their tragedy.

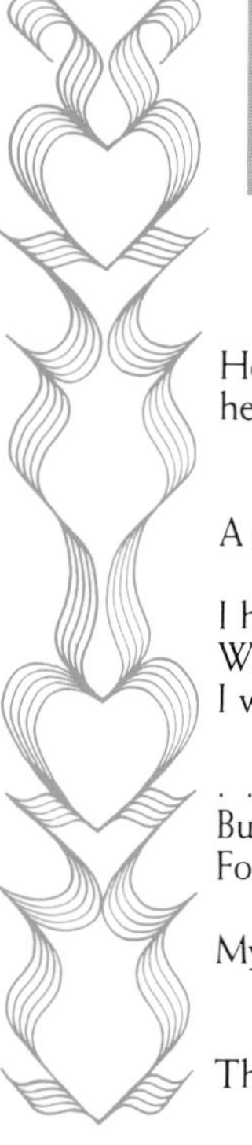

WHAT HIS HEART THINKS HIS TONGUE SPEAKS

A merry heart goes all the day. – Shakespeare

He hath a heart as sound as a bell, and his tongue is the clapper; for what his heart thinks his tongue speaks.

—*MUCH ADO ABOUT NOTHING*

A goodly apple rotten at the heart. —*MERCHANT OF VENICE*

I here do give thee that, with all my heart
Which, but thou hast already, with all my heart
I would keep from thee.

. . . 'Tis not long after
But I will wear my heart upon my sleeve
For daws to peck at.

My heart is turn'd to stone; I strike it, and it hurts my hand.

—*OTHELLO*

These words are razors to my wounded heart. —*TITUS ANDRONICUS*

Ferdinand: Here's my hand.
Miranda: And mine, with my heart in't. —*THE TEMPEST*

What infinite heart's ease
Must kings neglect that private men enjoy!

All offences, my lord, come from the heart; never came any from mine that might offend your majesty. —*HENRY V*

What stronger breastplate than a heart untainted! —2 *HENRY VI*

My crown is in my heart, not on my head.

O tiger's heart wrapp'd in a woman's hide! —3 *HENRY VI*

False face must hide what the false heart doth know. —*MACBETH*

Words, words, mere words, no matter from the heart.
—*TROILUS AND CRESSIDA*

So the heart be right, it is no matter which way the head lieth.
—Sir Walter Raleigh

The heart of man is of itself but little, yet great things cannot fill it: it is not big enough at one meal to satisfy a bird, and yet the whole world cannot satisfy it. —Thomas Dekker

Better a little chiding than a great deal of heartbreak.
—THE MERRY WIVES OF WINDSOR

. . . 'tis bitter cold
And I am sick at heart.

. . . Give me that man
That is not passion's slave, and I will wear him
In my heart's core, ay, in my heart of heart,
As I do thee.

Now cracks a noble heart. Good night, sweet prince . . .
—HAMLET

I have the heart and stomach of a king, and of a king of England too.
—Elizabeth I

When I am dead and opened, you shall find 'Calais' lying in my heart.
—Mary Tudor

A good heart is worth gold. – Shakespeare

The heart has its reasons which reason knows nothing of. . . . We know the truth, not only by the reason, but by the heart.
– Blaise Pascal

The heart is a brittle thing, and one false vow can break it.
– E.G. Bulwer-Lytton

A SHAKESPEAREAN CARDIOGRAPH

The graph below shows the number of times, according to the Oxford Shakespeare Concordances, *that Shakespeare used the word heart or a heart-like word (such as heartily, heartless) in each of his plays. The plays are listed chronologically from left to right.*

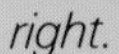

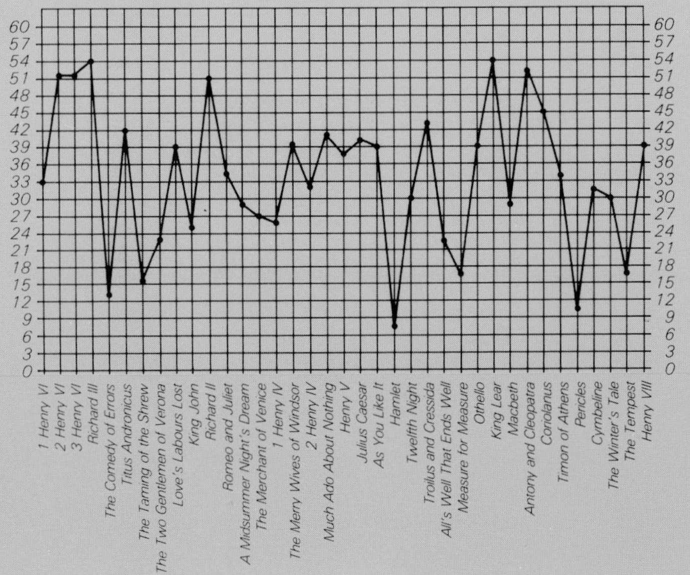

SHAKESPEARE'S SONNETS

The word *heart* is used 56 times in the 154 poems which make up Shakespeare's famous sonnet sequence. Eight occur in a single poem, Sonnet 46, in which Shakespeare weaves an elaborate metaphor of litigation in which the heart and the eye contend with one another for rights to the portrait of the young man (Herbert, Earl of Pembroke) who is the subject of the poem:

Mine eye and heart are at a mortal war,
How to divide the conquest of thy sight;
Mine eye my heart thy picture's sight would bar,
My heart mine eye the freedom of that right.
My heart doth plead that thou in him dost lie,
A closet never pierced with crystal eyes,
But the defendant [i.e., eye] doth that plea deny,
And says in him thy fair appearance lies.
To 'cide [decide] this title is impaneled
A quest [jury] of thoughts, all tenants to the heart;
And by their verdict is determined
The clear eye's moiety and the dear heart's part.
As thus; mine eye's due is thy outward part,
And my heart's right thy inward love of heart.

–William Shakespeare

Of its 56 appearances throughout the sonnets, the word *heart* appears in a rhyming position—that is, at the end of a line—only 17 times. On these euphonious occasions, it is made to rhyme with only three other words: *part* (10 times), *art* (6 times), *depart* (once). And speaking of rhymes, one contemporary poet's handbook lists 21 modern English words that rhyme with heart. Can you think of more than Shakespeare did?

"ENTER GIOVANNI WITH A HEART UPON HIS DAGGER"

The heart, both as concept and stage prop, is put to frequent use in many sensationalistic Renaissance plays. Elizabethan dramatist John Ford, author of The Broken Heart *and other grim and powerful plays, identified the heart with all the pleasurable and painful aspects of romantic love. It is mentioned repeatedly in many of his plays, but nowhere is it used more shockingly than in the tragedy* 'Tis Pity She's a Whore. *The play, first printed in 1633, was one of the most audacious of its time, concerning incestuous love.*

Annabella and Giovanni are of a noble family. Both are willful and passionate, and Giovanni gives signs throughout of a morbid, violent temperament. When Annabella becomes pregnant, and Giovanni learns that their affair has been discovered, he murders her. In the excerpt from the climax of the play printed below, Giovanni enters, carrying his sister's (and lover's) heart upon his dagger. The shock of the revelations kills their father Florio, and Giovanni dies after striking down Annabella's corrupt husband, Sorranzo.

Enter Giovanni with a heart upon his dagger

GIOVANNI. Here, here, Sorranzo! trimmed in reeking blood,
That triumphs over death, proud in the spoil
Of love and vengeance! Fate, or all the powers
That guide the motions of immortal souls,
Could not prevent me.

CARDINAL. What means this?

FLORIO. Son Giovanni!
GIOVANNI. Be not amazed: if your misgiving hearts
Shrink at an idle sight, what bloodless fear
Of coward passion would have seized your senses,
Had you beheld the rape of life and beauty
Which I have acted!
. . .'tis a heart,
A heart my lords, in which is mine entombed:
Tis Annabella's heart. . .
Have you all no faith
To credit yet my triumphs?
Here I swear
By all that you call sacred, by the love
I bore my Annabella whilst she lived,
These hands have from her bosom ripped this heart.
CARDINAL. Monster of children! see what thou hast done,
Broke thy old father's heart.

Two things are bad for the heart—running up stairs and running down people.
—Bernard M. Baruch

The hardest trial of the heart is, whether it can bear a rival's failure without truimph.
—Conrad Aiken

HEART-BURIAL

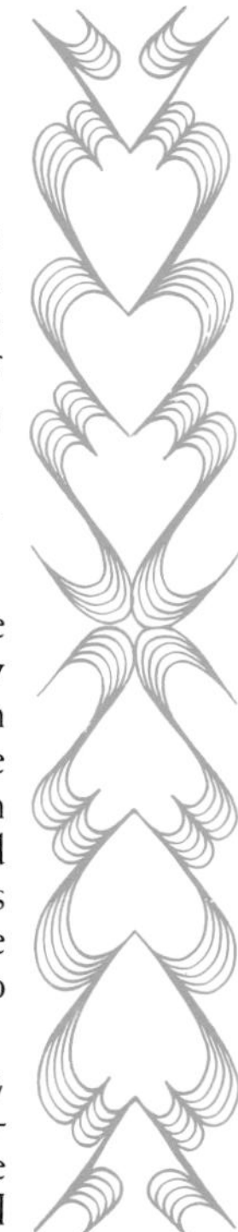

It was not the livers or brains or entrails of saints that were lifted from the body in sublimest autopsy, it was the heart, thus snipped and cradled into worshipful palms, then soaked in wine and herbs and set into silver reliquaries for the veneration of the faithful. It follows quite naturally that Love should choose such an organ for its bower. In the absence of Love, the canker gnaws it; when Love blooms therein, the heart dances and tremor cordis *is upon one.*

–Richard Selzer, M.D.

Burial of the heart apart from the body is a very ancient practice. The special reverence shown towards the heart is doubtless due to its early association with the soul of man, his affections, courage and conscience. In medieval Europe heart-burial was fairly common. Some of the more notable cases are those of Richard I, whose heart, preserved in a casket, was placed in Rouen cathedral; Henry III, buried in Normandy; Eleanor, queen of Edward I, in Lincoln; Edward I, in Jerusalem; Louis IX, Philip III, Louis XIII and Louis XIV, in Paris. Since the 17th century the hearts of deceased members of the house of Hapsburg have been buried apart from the body in the Loretto chapel in the Augustiner Kirche, Vienna.

Sometimes other parts of the body, removed in the process of embalming, are given separate and solemn burial. Thus the viscera of the popes from Sixtus V (1590) onward have been preserved in the parish church of the Quirinal. The custom of heart-burial was forbidden by Pope Boniface VIII (1294-1303), but Benedict XI withdrew the prohibition.

Robert Bruce wished his heart to rest in the church of the Holy Sepulchre in Jerusalem, and on his deathbed entrusted the fulfillment of his wish to Douglas, who broke his journey to join the Spaniards in their war with the Moorish king of Granada. He was killed in battle, the heart of Bruce enclosed in a silver casket hanging around his neck. Subsequently the heart was buried at Melrose Abbey.

The heart of James, marquess of Montrose, executed by the Scottish Covenanters in 1650, was recovered from his body, which had been buried by the roadside outside Edinburgh, and, enclosed in a steel box, was sent to the duke of Montrose, then in exile. It was lost on its journey, and years after-

THE HONORABLE HEART OF LA TOUR D'AUVERGNE

Among the proverbial landmarks in the life and death of French soldier La Tour d'Auvergne (b. 1743), the disposition of his courageous heart is not likely to be forgotten. After the heroic death of this "First Grenadier of France" in 1800, Napoleon Bonaparte led the entire French army in a three-day period of mourning. La Tour's surviving comrades in the military took up a collection to purchase a silver urn for the hero's heart. The prized vessel was for many years borne by the company of the 46th Grenadiers, who eventually entrusted it to Garibaldi. Eventually, in 1883, the noble heart was placed in the custody of the City of Paris.

wards was discovered in a curiosity shop in Flanders. Taken by a member of the Montrose family to India, it was stolen as an amulet by a native chief, was once more regained, and finally lost in France during the Revolution.

Among other notable 17th-century cases is that of James II, whose heart was buried in the church of the Convent of the Visitation at Chaillot near Paris, and that of Sir William Temple, at Moor Park, Farnham.

The last ceremonial burial of a heart in England was that of Paul Whitehead, secretary to the Monks of Medmenham club, in 1775, the interment taking place in the Le Despenser mausoleum at High Wycombe, Buckinghamshire.

Bury My Heart in Missolonghi

Ostracized from English society after scandal and controversy, Lord Byron—once the charismatic darling of the English Romantics—gave his heart to the cause of Greek liberty. He died in 1824, consummating a period of fervent and wholeheartedly exhaustive efforts on behalf of Greece's revolution against the Turks. General mourning among the Greek populace continued for 21 days. When Byron's body was eventually carried back to England, his heart, at the request of the Greek government, remained in the town of Missolonghi, the site of Byron's noblest actions. There, a small monument was raised to commemorate the heart that lay entombed beneath it.

Of later cases of heart-burial, the most notable are those of Daniel O'Connell, whose heart is at Rome, Shelley at Bournemouth, Louis XVII at Venice, Kosciusko at the Polish museum at Rapperschwyll, Lake Zurich, and the marquess of Bute, taken by his widow to Jerusalem for burial in 1900.

The Lost Heart

A Curious Historical Anecdote

We all of us lose our heart at least once in our lives—speaking metaphorically, of course. However, the heart of the Marquis of Montrose, preserved after he died, has been appearing and disappearing, passing from hand to hand, for over three hundred years.

The Marquis had the misfortune of having been on the losing side during the English Civil War. In 1650, he was first hanged, and then his body dismembered, the usual fate of those foolish or brave enough to oppose the prevailing power. The Napier family, having among their numbeı several Lords, were Montrose's most faithful friends. Montrose had often promised Lady Napier that when he died, she should have his heart. After the burial of the Marquis' body, a friend of the Napiers, under cover of darkness, exhumed the corpse and removed the heart. The organ was embalmed by a "skillful apothecary," wrapped in a coarse cloth, and placed in a small steel case fashioned from the blade of the Marquis' sword. This was in turn placed in a box made of gold and decorated with delicate filigree work, and then, box within box, was deposited in a hefty urn made of silver.

Lady Napier kept the urn for some time (indeed, it sat on a table by her bedside). She later sent it to the Marquis' son, then in exile on the continent. Although the young Marquis later returned to the British Isles, he apparently left the urn in the keeping of his good friend, the young Lord Napier, who had elected to stay in Europe. Soon after the friends parted, Lord Napier was robbed, and the golden box stolen.

It was assumed that the box would never be seen again, but in one of the many remarkable coincidences that mark the Montrose story, the box was discovered among the possessions of a collector in Holland—and by a close friend of the Napier family familiar with the story of the heart. He bought it and returned it to the Napiers. Almost a century later, the box and its contents passed into the possession of a Napier daughter, Hester. When she, her husband, and son took ship for India, where her husband had secured a job in the British administration, the golden casket went with them. En route, their ship was attacked by a French frigate (at that time, England and France were at war). Hester, her son and husband stayed on deck throughout the action. A shell from the frigate struck a gun, killed several men, and sprayed splinters across the deck. One splinter struck the bag in which Hester had collected all her valuables. The golden box was destroyed, but the steel container holding the heart was unscratched. In India, Hester's husband hired local goldsmiths to produce a replica of the box, on which the story of Montrose's life and death were engraved in several Indian dialects.

Unfortunately, the box and its contents soon acquired among the Indians the reputation of being a talisman so powerful that whoever possessed it could never be hurt in battle. Inevitably, the casket was stolen. Although it was rumored to have passed into the collection of a local maharajah, nothing could be done to prove this, or to regain it. Almost twenty years later, Hester's son Alexander had occasion to visit the prince reputed to own the box. During a hunt in which both men engaged, Alexander allowed the prince to kill a prize boar. In gratitude, the prince asked Alexander how he could demonstrate his appreciation. Alexander delicately introduced the story of the box and its contents. The prince admitted having bought the casket, at a great cost. However, he unhesitantly gave it up, and the heart was once again in the possession of the Napier family.

In 1792 Alexander and his parents set out to return to England. They traveled across France, and were just about to take ship from Boulogne for home when the Revolutionary government then in power passed a law requiring all gold and silver to be turned over to the state. It seemed impossible to smuggle the golden box past the port authorities, so Hester found an Englishwoman by the name of Knowles living quietly in Boulogne. The box and its contents were given into her possession, until such time as they could be reclaimed. While Hester and her family arrived safely home, any hopes of soon recovering the casket were dashed when war broke out between England and France. It was not until 1815, when a lasting peace was finally secured, that Alexander was able to make the short trip back to Boulogne to reclaim the Napier treasure. But Mrs. Knowles had died, and there was no record of the disposal of her possessions.

The box and its contents have not turned up since. Perhaps, this time, they are really gone, and the heart of Lord Montrose has been cast away on some alien ground. However, considering its unique record of reappearances, it is probably still premature to mark the story "closed." So, if, in a dusty, fly-specked window of some old curiosity shop, you catch sight of a dingy casket with strange writing upon it, go in and take it up. And if, inside, you find a steel container the shape and size of an egg, look further. If, in the steel egg, you find a packet wrapped in a rough cloth spread over with a substance like dried glue, it is likely that you are holding in your hands that elusive wandering heart of the Marquis of Montrose.

With every pleasing, every prudent part,
Say, what can Chloe want?—She wants a heart.
She speaks, behaves, and acts just as she ought;
But never, never, reached one generous thought.
Virtue she finds too painful an endeavour,
Content to dwell in decencies forever.
So very reasonable, so unmoved,
As never yet to love, or to be loved.
She, while her lover pants upon her breast,
Can mark the figures on an Indian chest;
And when she sees her friend in deep despair,
Observes how much a chintz exceeds mohair. . . .
Chloe is prudent—Would you too be wise?
Then never break your heart when Chloe dies.

—Alexander Pope

THE EXCHANGE

by Samuel Taylor Coleridge

We pledged our hearts, my love and I,—
I in my arms the maiden clasping;
I could not guess the reason why,
But, oh! I trembled like an aspen.

Her father's love she bade me gain;
I went, but shook like any reed!
I strove to act the man—in vain!
We had exchanged our hearts indeed.

The Heart That Would Not Burn

A common superstition among the Romans was the belief that the heart of a person who had been poisoned would not burn. This notion seems to have originated in India and been passed on to the Romans by the Syrians. Germanicus, governor of Syria during the reign of the Emperor Tiberius, died of a prolonged and undiagnosed illness in the year 19 A.D. When his rival and enemy, Piso, was brought to trial, one piece of evidence offered against him was the fact that after Germanicus had been cremated his heart was found whole and unsinged in the ashes.

Percy Bysshe Shelley, one of England's greatest Romantic poets, drowned at the age of 29 when his sailboat sank off the Italian coast in 1822.

Shelley's body was recovered and his closest friends, Lord Byron, Leigh Hunt, and Edward Trelawny, arranged to have it cremated. Trelawny's record of the ceremony notes that the fire was fierce, and consumed all of the body but the heart, which he snatched from the flames, severely burning his hand. Leigh Hunt prevailed upon Trelawny to give up the heart, but he in turn was persuaded to turn it over to Shelley's wife, Mary (the author of *Frankenstein*). Mary never remarried, and through her long life, the heart was always with her. Wrapped in silk, it was kept in a special pouch attached to one of Shelley's volumes of poetry. After her death, it was eventually buried with the body of one of their sons.

HEART'S COMPASS

by Dante Gabriel Rossetti

Sometimes thou seem'st not as thyself alone,
But as the meaning of all things that are;
A breathless wonder, shadowing forth afar
Some heavenly solstice hushed and halcyon,
Whose unstirred lips are music's visible tone,
Whose eyes the sun-gate of the soul unbar,
Being of its furthest fires oracular—
The evident heart of all life sown and mown.
Even such love is; and is not thy name Love?
Yea, but thy hand the Love-god rends apart
All gathering clouds of Night's ambiguous art,
Flings them far down, and sets thine eyes above;
And simply, as some gage of flower or glove,
Stakes with a smile the world against thy heart.

MY HEART IS A LUTE

by Anne Barnard

Alas, that my heart is a lute,
Whereon you have learned to play!
For a many years it was mute,
Until one summer's day
You took it, and touched it, and made it thrill,
And it thrills and throbs, and quivers still!

I had known you, dear, so long!
Yet my heart did not tell me why
It should burst one morn into song,
And wake to new life with a cry,
Like a babe that sees the light of the sun,
And for whom this great world has just begun.

Your lute is enshrined, cased in,
Kept close with love's magic key,
So no hand but yours can win
And wake it to minstrelsy;
Yet leave it not silent too long, nor alone,
Lest the strings should break, and the music be done.

My heart leaps up when I behold
A rainbow in the sky:
So was it when my life began;
So is it now I am a man;
So be it when I shall grow old,
Or let me die!
The Child is father of the Man;
And I could wish my days to be
Bound each to each by natural piety.

—William Wordsworth

My heart's in the Highlands, my heart is not here,
My heart's in the Highlands, a-chasing the deer;
A-chasing the wild deer, and following the roe,
My heart's in the Highlands wherever I go.

—Robert Burns

When the voices of children are heard on the green
And laughing is heard on the hill,
My heart is at rest within my breast
And everything else is still.

—William Blake

But O heart! heart! heart!
O the bleeding drops of red,
Where on the deck my Captain lies
Fallen cold and dead.

—Walt Whitman

The happiest heart that ever beat
Was in some quiet breast
That found the common daylight sweet,
And left to Heaven the rest.

—John V. Cheney

The Mind lives on the Heart
Like any Parasite—
If that is full of Meat
The Mind is fat.

But if the Heart omit
Emaciate the Wit—
The Aliment of it
So absolute.

—Emily Dickinson

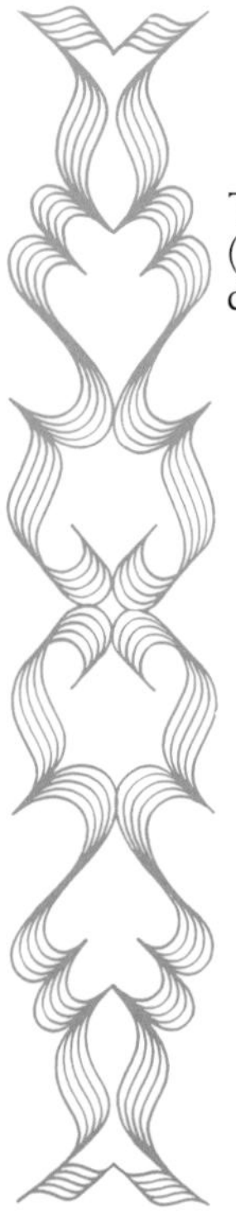

LITERARY QUIZ

The title poem of W.D. Snodgrass's Pulitzer Prize-winning book *Heart's Needle* (1959) was adapted from the old Irish saying that "An only daughter is the needle of the heart." Can you match the poets with the hearty quotes below?

a. Charlotte Bronte
b. Lewis Carroll
c. Emily Dickinson
d. John Keats
e. Andrew Marvell
f. Homer
g. George Gordon, Lord Byron
h. John Donne
i. William Shakespeare
j. Percy Shelley
k. Sir John Suckling
l. William Butler Yeats
m. Robert Browning
n. Henry Wadsworth Longfellow
o. Alfred, Lord Tennyson

1. *When the heart is on fire, some sparks fly out of the mouth.*
2. *An age at least to every part*
   And the last age should show your heart.
3. *Batter my heart, three-personed God . . .*
4. *Ah, nothing is too late,*
   Till the tired heart shall cease to palpitate.
5. *A pity beyond all telling*
   Is hid in the heart of love.

6. *There is no instinct like that of the heart.*

7. *My heart aches, and a drowsiness numbness pains*
   My sense, as though of hemlock I had drunk. . . .

8. *It is not, nor it cannot come to good,*
   But break my heart, for I must hold my tongue.

9. *Never morning wore to evening, but some heart did break.*

10. *The human heart has hidden treasures,*
    In secret kept, in silence sealed.

11. *Open my heart, and you will see*
    Graved inside of it, "Italy."

12. *One by one, and two by two,*
    He toss'd them human hearts to chew.

13. *I prithee send me back my heart,*
    Since I cannot have thine;
    For if from yours you will not part,
    Why then shouldst thou have mine?

14. *The mind lives on the heart*
    Like any parasite.

15. *And my heart is like nothing so much as a bowl*
    Brimming over with quivering curds.

Answers:
1–f, 2–e, 3–h, 4–n, 5–l, 6–g, 7–d, 8–i, 9–o, 10–a, 11–m, 12–j, 13–k, 14–c, 15–b.

Now, can you match the titles of the following literary works with their authors?

	Title		Author
1.	*The Heart Keeper*	a.	Nathaniel West
2.	*The Heart of Man*	b.	Conrad Aiken
3.	*The Heart of Midlothain*	c.	Carson McCullers
4.	*In the Heart of the Heart of the Country*	d.	Françoise Sagan
5.	*Hearts of the West*	e.	Mikhail Bulgakov
6.	*The Heart of the Matter*	f.	Dee Brown
7.	*Heartbreak House*	g.	Joseph Conrad
8.	*Heart of Darkness*	h.	Erich Fromm
9.	*The Heart Is a Lonely Hunter*	i.	Belasco & Hearne
10.	*The Heart of a Dog*	j.	Sir Walter Scott
11.	*A Heart for the Gods of Mexico*	k.	Graham Greene
12.	*Bury My Heart at Wounded Knee*	l.	George Bernard Shaw
13.	*Hearts of Oak*	m.	William Gass
14.	*Miss Lonelyhearts*	n.	O. Henry

Answers: 1-d, 2-h, 3-j, 4-m, 5-n, 6-k, 7-l, 8-g, 9-c, 10-e, 11-b, 12-f, 13-i, 14-a.

The Queen of Hearts, she made some tarts
All on a summer's day;
The Knave of Hearts, he stole the tarts
And took them clean away.

–Mother Goose

HEARTS & PLAYING CARDS

With spots quadrangular of diamond form,
Ensanguined hearts, clubs typical of strife,
And spades, the emblem of untimely graves.

—William Cowper

Using spades, diamonds, clubs, and hearts to identify the four suits is now widespread, but it was not always so. Before these won out, a remarkably diverse—and sometimes bizarre—assortment of symbols was featured.

The first recorded use of playing cards was in the Orient in the 12th century. How long they had existed before and precisely where they were developed are unknown. Very early Chinese decks featured coins in varying numbers to denote each suit. Such cards were probably used simply for amusement.

The first cards to reach Europe had an ostensibly more serious purpose. These "Tarot" cards, used as a fortune-telling aid, were introduced in the 12th century. There may have been 50 or more cards to a deck, all featuring hand-painted allegorical scenes. Wealthy merchants and nobles commissioned well-known artists to paint Tarot decks for them, and each was a unique work of art. Indeed, because each deck had to be painted by hand, only the wealthy could afford them. The introduction of the printing press gradually changed all that: By the 16th century, cards had become a familiar sight, widely available and very popular.

No longer used simply for divination or for show, cards had become the basis of a number of games. Just when and how this happened is unclear, although evidence shows that many card games were widely known as early as the 14th century. Indeed, even though cards were still very expensive, the market for them was large enough for England and some Italian city-states to enforce embargoes forbidding importers from bringing in the handsome decks produced in Germany, because native cardmakers were being driven out of business by the competition.

Because each cardmaker favored his own symbols and ideas, literally hundreds were used to represent the four suits—everything from mythological beasts to wild animals to acorns. Even the number of cards in a deck fluctuated. The advent of the printing press helped bring a certain uniformity to the field: playing cards became more and more standardized, with fewer individual quirks.

A French knight brought even more uniformity to the field when, in the 16th century, he invented the "modern" deck of cards in which the four suits are represented by hearts, diamonds (or squares), clovers, and pikeheads. The heart had been used as early as the 14th century as a symbol for one of the suits. That it should have endured is not surprising—it is a universal symbol, immediately recognizable, and its simplicity lends itself well to the design of a deck of cards.

The English enthusiastically adopted the French deck and in the process further simplified the symbols into today's spades, hearts, diamonds, and clubs. Cards quickly became popular entertainment among all levels of society. This is testified to by the fact that as early as 1633 some miscreant New England Puritans were caught in a game of cards and fined the stiff sum of two pounds each for their moral lapse.

GAME OF HEARTS

The game of Hearts was developed in the 1920s. Since then, some 20 different variations on the basic game—such as Joker Hearts, Match Style Hearts, Greek Hearts, and Progressive Hearts—have been developed. Basic rules for the most popular version of Hearts—known as Black Queen, Slippery Anne, or Discard Hearts—are fairly simple, and the most important one to remember is that in Hearts the person with the lowest *score wins.*

A standard pack of cards (minus jokers) is used, and from three to six people may play. The cards are shuffled and dealt so that each player has the same number. Any left over are placed face down in the center of the table and must be collected by the first person to take a heart. Before play begins, each player selects three cards from his hand and passes them, face down, to the player on his left. A player must pass before he can look at the cards he has received from his neighbor.

The player who has been dealt the two of clubs makes the opening lead; the other players must play cards of the same suit. If they are unable to follow suit, they may discard from any of the others. The ace is high in all suits, with the rest of the cards descending in value in the usual order. The person who has played the highest card in the suit that was led must take the hand.

The object is to avoid taking any hearts, since each heart counts one point. Players also try to avoid the queen of spades, worth 13 points. On the other hand, a daring player with the right hand can attempt to take all the hearts and *the queen of spades. If he succeeds all the players receive twenty-six points and he receives none.*

No standard number of points constitutes a game, and any number of deals may be played before the players agree to stop and add up the score. At that point, players' individual totals may be combined into a grand total which is then divided by the number of players to determine an average score. Each player who has scored above the average pays into the pot the difference between this average and his own score. Each player having a total score below the average collects the difference between that score and his own from the pot.

HEARTS WITH DICE, OR, DICE WITH HEARTS

Sometimes called "hearts due," this game of hearts is designed for two or more players using six ordinary dice. Dice marked with letters spelling "HEARTS" may also be used, although this is now uncommon.

After preliminary rolls to select the first shooter (usually simply the highest scorer), players each roll the six dice once and tally up their scores. Points are awarded as follows:

1 (H)-5 points
1,2 (H,E)-10 points
1,2,3 (H,E,A)-15 points
1,2,3,4 (H,E,A,R)-20 points
1,2,3,4,5 (H,E,A,R,T)-25 points
1,2,3,4,5,6 (H,E,A,R,T,S)-35 points

Play may be limited to one round, or extended to any number of rounds previously agreed upon. The winner may be either the highest scorer or the first to reach a set total, whichever the players prefer.

When a double (two dice showing the same value) or triple appears in a throw, only one will count. If, however, a player throws three 1's (or H's), he loses all points and must start over.

You Will Meet A Tall, Warm-Hearted Stranger

Since Tarot decks are the ancestors of today's playing cards, it's not surprising that some psychics prefer to use a regular deck of playing cards when they attempt to read the future.

The cards are shuffled and then arranged in a pattern similar to that used in a traditional Tarot reading. Although it's been said that the cards only focus the seer's energies and don't in themselves carry a message, various systems have been worked out so that anyone can "read" the cards' meanings—and their interpretations are sometimes quite at variance.

Cards say different things depending on how they come out of the deck. A king, for instance, has one meaning if it's right side up, another if it's upside down, or reversed.

Bearing all this in mind, here are some messages your hearts might be sending you.

ACE Untroubled family life.
Reversed: Quarrelsome, difficult family life.

KING A fair-haired, easygoing man will have an influence in your future.
Reversed: In your future there is an exacting individual who is difficult to get along with.

QUEEN A fair-haired woman, virtuous and true, will have some part in your life.
Reversed: Trouble lies ahead in the path of love.

JACK A loyal, kindly young man will be involved in your life.
Reversed: Loyal, kind-hearted thoughts directed at you, or directed outward by you.

TEN A symbol of one's work and/or of love.
Reversed: An unexpected and pleasant event is likely.

NINE Success. A harmonious life. Contentment.
Reversed: Obstacles or worries will block your path.

EIGHT An unexpected visit or present is likely.
Reversed: An auburn-haired young woman will be connected in some pleasant way with your future.

SEVEN Thoughts of a loved one are with you.
Reversed: The hopes and desires of a loved one will influence your course of action.

OF DREAMS AND THE HEART

While Sigmund Freud reports that hollow boxes or baskets in certain dreams may represent the heart, Zolar's Encyclopedia and Dictionary of Dreams *tells us just what to expect from the appearances of the heart in our dreams. A dream in which you are eating heart meat, Zolar declares, portends a happy love affair; and to dream of cooking heart meat signifies a successful future. Should you dream of losing your heart, it's not a romance—it means that death is near. Dreaming of having a wounded heart relates to marital separation, while dreaming of the heart of an unmarried person suggests elopement and marriage. And those of our readers plagued by dreams of being breathless due to heart trouble, should take heart—Zolar says it means you will surpass your friends.*

ANATOMY OF THE HEART

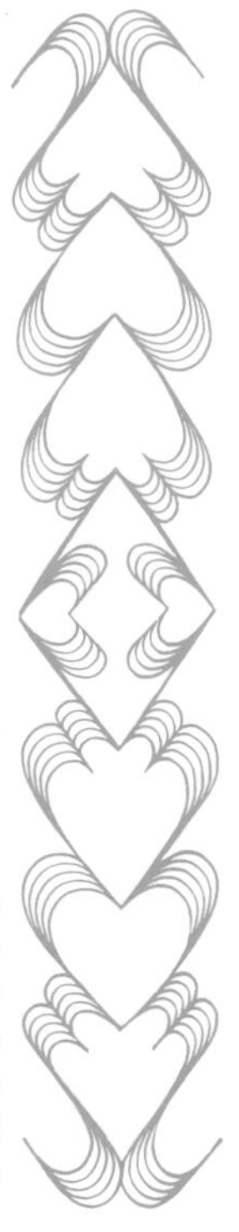

According to Aristotle, the hearts of horses and some breeds of oxen contained a bone that provided support for the organ.

The Greek physician Galen, born in 130 A.D., is remembered primarily for his extensive theoretical writings on medicine and the human body. Much of his knowledge of anatomy was gathered first-hand during the time he served as physician to the gladiators who performed in the city of Pergamon.

Galen treated many gladiators who had been wounded in the heart. While such injuries were invariably fatal, some of the men might linger on for as long as a day and a night. Galen wrote that these men retained their senses until the end, thus refuting the belief, passed down from the Sumerians, that the heart was the seat of man's intelligence.

Sixteenth century French satirist François Rabelais was also noted as a doctor. His statements about the heart conform with the prevailing scientific views of his time. In *Pantagruel* he writes:

The heart doth in its left-side ventricle so thinnify the blood, that it thereby obtains the name of spiritual; which being sent through the arteries to all the members of the body, serveth to warm, and winnow, or fan the other blood which runneth through the veins. The lights never cease with its lappets and bellows to cool and refresh it; in acknowledgment of which good the heart, through the arterial vein, imparts unto it the choicest of its blood. At last it is made so fine and subtle within the rete mirabile, that thereafter those animal spirits are framed and composed of it; by means whereof the imagination, discourse, judgment, resolution, deliberation, ratiocination and memory have their rise, actings, and operations.

A Modern Definition

The human heart is divided by a septum into two halves, right and left, each half being further constricted into two cavities, the upper of the two being termed the auricle *[atrium] and the lower the* ventricle. *The heart therefore consists of four chambers or cavities, two forming the right half, the right auricle and right ventricle, and two the left half, the left auricle and left ventricle. The right half of the heart contains venous or impure blood; the left, arterial or pure blood. From the cavity of the left ventricle the pure blood is carried into a large artery, the* aorta, *through the numerous branches of which it is distributed to all parts of the body, with the exception of the lungs. In its passage through the capillaries of the body the blood gives up to the tissues the materials necessary for their growth and nourishment, and at the same time receives from the tissues the waste products resulting from their metabolism, and in doing so becomes changed from arterial or pure blood into venous or impure blood, which is collected by the veins and through them returned to the right auricle of the heart. From this cavity the impure blood passes into the right ventricle, from which it is conveyed through the* pulmonary arteries *to the lungs. In the capillaries of the lungs it again becomes arterialized, and is then carried to the left auricle by the* pulmonary veins. *From this cavity it passes into that of the left ventricle, from which the cycle once more begins.*

–Henry Gray, M.D., F.R.S.,
from the Unabridged Running Press
Edition of *Gray's Anatomy,* 1901

An advantage of having a hard heart is that it will take a lot to break it.

–W. Burton Baldry

HEARTBROKEN

Some leisurely paging through Stedman's Medical Dictionary *will yield the following assortment of hearts:*

Armored heart: *calcareous deposits in the pericardium occurring in subacute or chronic inflammation.*

Beer-heart: *a hypertrophied heart supposedly due to the greater load resulting from an excessive consumption of fluids.*

Bony heart: *the presence of more or less extensive calcareous patches in the pericardium and walls of the heart.*

Forward heart failure: *the theory of forward failure maintains that the phenomena of congestive heart failure result from the inadequate cardiac output, and especially from the consequent inadequacy of renal blood flow with resulting retention of sodium and water.*

Hairy heart: *pericarditis in which the heart is seen post mortem to be covered with a shaggy, fibrinous exudate; cor hirsutum; cor tomentosum; trichocardia; shaggy pericardium.*

Heart hurry: *rapid action of the heart; tachycardia.*

Icing heart: *pericarditis in which the heart is seen post mortem covered with a thick, white coat like the icing of cake.*

Irritable heart: *soldier's heart; neurocirculatory asthenia; a cardiac neurosis marked by rapid pulse, dyspnea, and various anxiety symptoms, associated with an increased susceptibility to fatigue.*

Skin heart: *the peripheral blood vessels.*

Tiger heart: *a fatty degenerated heart in which the fat is disposed in the form of broken stripes.*

Tobacco heart: *cardiac irritability marked by irregular action, palpitation, and sometimes pain, occurring as a result of the excessive use of tobacco.*

Waist of the heart: *in the chest x-ray, the middle segment of the cardiac silhouette, containing the pulmonary salient.*

THE WORLD'S LARGEST VALENTINE

For more than 30 years, Philadelphia's Franklin Institute has had the distinction of being a cultural and educational institution that actually has a heart. Built in 1953, the museum's famous walk-through model of a human heart is 28 feet wide and 18 feet high—almost 15,000 times larger than a human heart. Accompanied by a recording of the sounds of a beating heart, visitors travel the route a blood corpuscle takes as it pumps through the heart. Along the way, they can see and touch larger-than-life reproductions of the strategic parts of the organ.

To construct the giant heart, designers used cross sections of frozen beef hearts to produce drawings that were projected on plywood and cut out in concentric, interlocking rings. These were hooked together using 4,000 square feet of metal lath and 4 tons of papier-mâché. The exhibit was originally intended to be only a temporary structure, but from its unveiling it has drawn such crowds that it has never been dismantled. Now, 30 years and more than 10 million visitors later, the Franklin Institute has completed a $100,000 heart rehabilitation program.

Milestones in the Study of The Heart

When I first gave my mind to vivisection, as a means of discovering the motions and uses of the heart, and sought to discover these from actual inspection, and not from writings of others, I found the task so truly arduous, so full of difficulties, that I was almost tempted to think, with Fracastorius, that the motion of the heart was only to be comprehended by God. —William Harvey

1628
Circulation of the Blood through the body was described by William Harvey, an English physician.

1706
The Structure of the Left Ventricle and Distribution of Coronary Vessels were described by Raymond de Vieussens, a French anatomy professor.

1733
Blood Pressure was measured by Stephen Hales, an English clergyman and scientist.

1785
Digitalis, in the form of foxglove leaves, was introduced by English physician William Withering.

1816
The Stethoscope was invented by Rene T.H. Laennec, a French physician.

1893
The Atrioventricular Bundle, a muscle bundle connecting the right atrium with the ventricles of the heart, was discovered by Swiss anatomist Wilhelm His, Jr. It is also called the *bundle of His.*

1903
The Electrocardiograph, for showing the heart's electrical activity, was developed by Willem Einthoven, a Dutch physiologist.

1904
The Effect of Rheumatic Fever on the heart was described by German pathologist Ludwig Aschoff.

1905
The First "Successful" Heart Transplant: both donor and recipient were dogs. After the completed operation, the transplanted heart beat for one hour.

1908
Congenital Heart Disease was described and classified by Maude Abbott, a Canadian physician.

1912
First Diagnosis of Coronary Thrombosis and description of heart disease resulting from hardening of the arteries were made by James B. Herrick, an American cardiologist.

1930
Modern Method of Electrocardiology was developed by Frank N. Wilson, an American physician.

1944
First Surgery for Blue Babies was performed by Alfred Blalock, an American surgeon, and Helen B. Taussig, an American cardiologist.

1948
First Successful Operations for rheumatic heart disease were performed independently by Charles P. Bailey and Dwight E. Harken, American surgeons.

1951
Plastic Ball Valve for a leaky aortic (semilunar) valve was developed by American surgeon Charles Hufnagel.

1952
Open Heart Surgery was first successfully performed by F. John Lewis, an American surgeon. He used ice to lower body temperature and slow circulation so the heart remained dry during surgery.

1953
Mechanical Heart and Blood Purifier was used successfully for the first time by American surgeon John H. Gibbon.

1954
Human Cross-Circulation, permitting a second person's heart and lungs to pump the blood of a person under surgery, was developed by American surgeon C. Walton Lillehei.

1961
External Cardiac Massage, to restart a stopped heart without surgery, was introduced by J.R. Jude, an American cardiologist, and his associates.

1962
Cardioversion, a method of correcting fibrillation and irregular heartbeat by electric shock, was introduced by American cardiologist B. Lown.

1965
Assisting Hearts, mechanical devices to help a diseased or overworked left ventricle, were first successfully implanted by Michael E. DeBakey, and by Adrian Kantrowitz, American surgeons.

1967
First Transplant of a whole heart from one person to another was performed on Louis Washkansky, 55, at the Groote Schuur Hospital in Capetown, South Africa on December 3, 1967. In a five-hour operation, Dr. Christiaan Barnard and a team of 30 replaced Washkansky's heart with that of Denise Ann Darvall, 25. Washkansky died 18 days later.

1974
First Implantation of a donor heart without removing the patient's own heart was performed by a surgical team headed by Christiaan Barnard.

1980
Permanent Artificial Heart Implanted in calf at University of Utah Medical Center. This success encouraged surgeons to seek permission for implantation in human subject.

1982
First Implantation of Permanent Artificial Heart in a human being.

THE HEART-LUNG MACHINE

Newsweek *magazine (May 8, 1978) reported that John Wayne received the mitral valve of a pig's heart to replace a defective valve in his heart. Convalescing from open-heart surgery, Wayne remarked, "I feel like a new man. When I wake up in the morning and it's raining, I feel like rolling in the mud."*

Open-heart surgery, while never routine, is regularly and safely carried out many thousands of times each year. But until quite recently, there was no way surgeons could operate on the heart and still maintain its vital functions. Blood must circulate constantly through the body. If the supply of oxygenated blood to the brain is interrupted for as little as four minutes, permanent damage will result.

Designs for a machine that could assume all the heart's functions for short periods of time had been put forward as early as 1885, but the technology to carry them out simply didn't exist. Not until 1954, following some 19 years of research and development spearheaded by Dr. John Gibbon, was the first successful heart-lung machine produced. While the machine is functioning, the surgeon can work uninterrupted on the exposed heart, taking his time to carry out delicate repair work.

The heart-lung machine makes possible a complete cardiopulmonary bypass—all essential functions of the heart are assumed by the machine. Blood returning to the heart is diverted by means of plastic tubes in the two major veins (the venae cavae) responsible for returning blood to the heart. Blood reaching these veins is immediately shunted into the artificial "lung," where carbon dioxide is removed and oxygen is added to the blood. Then the blood is returned to the body via one of the arteries. A pump in the machine supplies just the right pressure to keep the blood circulating at the correct rate.

THE ARTIFICIAL HEART

On December 2, 1982, a surgical team headed by William C. De Vries, M.D., at the University of Utah Medical Center implanted the device, powered by six-foot hoses tethered to an air compressor the size of a shopping cart. Dr. Chase N. Peterson, vice president of health affairs for the University, described the operation as "something that is as exciting and thrilling as has ever been accomplished in medicine." The recipient, 61-year-old Dr. Barney B. Clark, lived 112 days.

Known as Jarvik-7 after its designer, Dr. Robert K. Jarvik, the artificial heart was the culmination of 25 years of development. In 1952, a mechanical heart crafted by General Motors took over for the heart of a patient for 50 minutes during surgery. In 1957, Dr. Tetsuzo Akutsu and Dr. Willem J. Kolff—now at the University of Utah Division of Artificial Organs and Dr. Jarvik's mentor—succeeded in keeping dogs alive for a matter of hours with a totally artificial implant. Jarvik-7, whose designer is also a sculptor, was the latest in a series first created in 1972. Made largely of molded polyurethane, it is slightly larger than a human heart but weighs about the same. Its cost: $16,450.

During the 7½-hour operation, performed to the beat of Ravel's "Bolero," two-thirds of Dr. Clark's diseased heart was removed, and Jarvik-7 was anchored to the left and right remaining chambers. A soft clicking sound was audible through the patient's chest as Jarvik-7 beat at a steady rate of 95 times per minute.

With the artificial heart, the possibility of rejection does not exist, since there is no foreign tissue to trigger the body's immune system. For nearly four months, except for when a defective valve had to be replaced, Jarvik-7 beat flawlessly. When the deterioration of Dr. Clark's other organs caused his death, the sturdy plastic heart was still going strong.

REFLECTIONS ON HEART TRANSPLANTS

"The reality of organ transplants," writes Dr. Shelby D. Gerking, "forces our society to focus on issues that before had been only aimless speculations. Unlike other organs, such as the kidney, the heart is an unpaired structure with little likelihood that the transplant will be made between two individuals in the same family where the immune response is less violent. This situation drastically reduces the number of options open to the surgeon and places him in the unenviable position of choosing the recipient and the donor. The heart of the recipient, while still partially functional, must be judged to be damaged beyond repair; the heart of the donor must be excised immediately after a fatal accident to safeguard the tissue from injury during the interim between removal and transplant. The quick removal of the donor heart has, according to some, demanded a substitution for cardiac arrest as a criterion of death. Our minds are so thoroughly conditioned to equate life with the beating heart that the possibility of using such a heart for transplantation calls into question the very foundations of our legal, moral, and ethical codes. For the time being, we can avoid this confrontation, but the search continues for some method of immobilizing the antibody-producing systems and even constructing a mechanical heart that can be implanted in place of the real thing. As long as man fears death, he will search for ways of prolonging life beyond his appointed years."

What the heart has once owned and had, it shall never lose. –H.W. Beecher

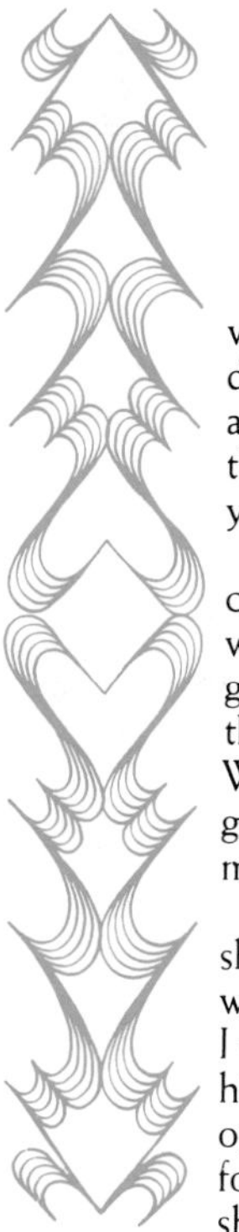

THE TELL-TALE HEART

by Edgar Allan Poe

True!—nervous—very, very dreadfully nervous I had been and am; but why *will* you say that I am mad? The disease had sharpened my senses—not destroyed—not dulled them. Above all was the sense of hearing acute. I heard all things in the heaven and in the earth. I heard many things in hell. How, then, am I mad? Hearken! and observe how healthily—how calmly I can tell you the whole story.

It is impossible to say how first the idea entered my brain; but, once conceived, it haunted me day and night. Object there was none. Passion there was none. I loved the old man. He had never wronged me. He had never given me insult. For his gold I had no desire. I think it was his eye! yes, it was this! He had the eye of a vulture—a pale blue eye, with a film over it. Whenever it fell upon me, my blood ran cold; and so by degrees—very gradually—I made up my mind to take the life of the old man, and thus rid myself of the eye forever.

Now this is the point. You fancy me mad. Madmen know nothing. But you should have seen *me*. You should have seen how wisely I proceeded—with what caution—with what foresight—with what dissimulation I went to work! I was never kinder to the old man than during the whole week before I killed him. And every night, about midnight, I turned the latch of his door and opened it—oh, so gently! And then, when I had made an opening sufficient for my head, I first put in a dark lantern, all closed, closed, so that no light shone out, and then I thrust in my head. Oh, you would have laughed to see how cunningly I thrust it in! I moved it slowly—very, very slowly, so that I might not disturb the old man's sleep. It took me an hour to place my whole head within the opening so far that I could see the old man as he lay upon his bed. Ha!—would a madman have been so wise as this? And then, when my head was well in the room, I undid the lantern cautiously—oh, so cautiously (for the hinges creaked) —I undid it just so much that a single thin ray fell upon the vulture eye. And this I did for seven long nights—every night just at midnight—but I found the eye always closed; and so it was impossible to do the work; for it was not the old man who vexed me, but his Evil Eye. And every morning, when the day broke, I went boldly into his chamber, and spoke courageously to him, calling him by name in a hearty tone, and inquiring how he had passed the night. So you see he would have been a very profound old man, indeed, to suspect that every night, just at twelve, I looked in upon him while he slept.

Upon the eighth night I was more than usually cautious in opening the door. A watch's minute hand moves more quickly than did mine. Never, before that night, had I *felt* the extent of my own powers—of my sagacity. I could scarcely contain my feelings of triumph. To think that there I was, opening the door, little by little, and the old man not even to dream of my secret deeds or thoughts. I fairly chuckled at the idea; and perhaps the old man heard me; for he moved in the bed suddenly, as if startled. Now you may think that I drew back—but no. His room was as black as pitch with the thick darkness, (for the shutters were close fastened, through fear of robbers,) and so I knew that he could not see the opening of the door, and I kept on pushing it steadily, steadily.

I had got my head in, and was about to open the lantern, when my thumb slipped upon the tin fastening, and the old man sprang up in the bed, crying out—"Who's there?"

I kept quite still and said nothing. For another hour I did not move a muscle, and in the meantime I did not hear the old man lie down. He was still sitting up in the bed, listening;—just as I have done, night after night, hearkening to the death-watches in the wall.

Presently I heard a slight groan, and I knew that it was the groan of mortal terror. It was not a groan of pain or of grief—oh, no!—it was the low stifled sound that arises from the bottom of the soul when overcharged with *awe*. I knew the sound well. Many a night, just at midnight, when all the world slept, it has welled up from my own bosom, deepening, with its dreadful echo, the terrors that distracted me. I say I knew it well. I knew what the old man felt, and pitied him, although I chuckled at heart. I knew that he had been lying awake ever since the first slight noise, when he had turned in the bed. His fears had been ever since growing upon him. He had been trying to fancy them causeless, but could not. He had been saying to himself—"It is nothing but the wind in the chimney—it is only a mouse crossing the floor," or "it is merely a cricket which has made a single chirp." Yes, he had been trying to comfort himself with these suppositions: but he had found all in vain. *All in vain;* because Death, in approaching the old man, had stalked with his black shadow before him, and the shadow had now reached and enveloped the victim. And it was the mournful influence of the unperceived shadow that caused him to feel—although he neither saw nor heard me—to *feel* the presence of my head within the room.

When I had waited a long time, very patiently, without hearing the old man lie down, I resolved to open a little—a very, very little crevice in the lantern. So I opened it—you cannot imagine how stealthily, stealthily—until, at length, a single dim ray, like the thread of the spider, shot from out the crevice and fell full upon the vulture eye.

It was open—wide, wide open—and I grew furious as I gazed upon it. I saw it with perfect distinctness—all a dull blue, with a hideous veil over it that chilled the very marrow in my bones; but I could see nothing else of the old man's face or person: for I had directed the ray as if by instinct, precisely upon the damned spot.

And now—have I not told you that what you mistake for madness is but over acuteness of the senses?—now, I say, there came to my ears *a low, dull, quick sound—much such a sound as a watch makes when enveloped in cotton.* I knew *that* sound well, too. It was the beating of the old man's heart. It increased my fury, as the beating of a drum stimulates the soldier into courage.

But even yet I refrained and kept still. I scarcely breathed. I held the lantern motionless. I tried how steadily I could maintain the ray upon the eye. Meantime the hellish tattoo of the heart increased. It grew quicker, and louder and louder every instant. The old man's terror *must* have been extreme! It grew louder, I say, louder every moment!—do you mark me well? I have told you that I am nervous: so I am. And now at the dead hour of the night, and amid the dreadful silence of that old house, so strange a noise as this excited me to uncontrollable wrath. Yet, for some minutes longer I refrained and kept still. But the beating grew louder, *louder*! I thought the heart must burst. And now a new anxiety seized me—the sound would be heard by a neighbor! The old man's hour had come! With a loud yell, I threw open the lantern and leaped into the room. He shrieked once—once only. In an instant I dragged him to the floor, and pulled the heavy bed over him. I then sat upon the bed and smiled gaily, to find the deed so far done. But, for many minutes, the heart beat on with a muffled sound. This, however, did not vex me; it would not be heard through the walls. At length it ceased. The old man was dead. I removed the bed and examined the corpse. Yes, he was stone, stone dead. I placed my hand upon the heart and held it there many minutes. There was no pulsation. The old man was stone dead. His eye would trouble *me* no more.

If still you think me mad, you will think so no longer when I describe the wise precautions I took for the concealment of the body. The night waned, and I worked hastily, but in silence. First of all I dismembered the corpse. I cut off the head and the arms and the legs.

I then took up three planks from the flooring of the chamber, and deposited all between the scantlings. I then replaced the boards so cleverly, so cunningly, that no human eye—not even *his*—could have detected anything wrong. There was nothing to wash out—no stain of any kind—no blood-spot whatever. I had been too wary for that. A tub had caught all—ha! ha!

When I had made an end of these labors, it was four o'clock—still dark as midnight. As the bell sounded the hour, there came a knocking at the street door. I went down to open it with a light heart,—for what had I *now* to fear? There entered three men, who introduced themselves, with perfect suavity, as officers of the police. A shriek had been heard by a neighbor during the night; suspicion of foul play had been aroused; information had been lodged at the police office, and they (the officers) had been deputed to search the premises.

I smiled,—for *what* had I to fear? I bade the gentlemen welcome. The shriek, I said, was my own in a dream. The old man, I mentioned, was absent in the country. I took my visiters all over the house. I bade them search—search *well*. I led them, at length, to *his* chamber. I showed them his treasures, secure, undisturbed. In the enthusiasm of my confidence, I brought chairs into the room, and desired them *here* to rest from their fatigues, while I myself, in the wild audacity of my perfect triumph, placed my own seat upon the very spot beneath which reposed the corpse of the victim.

The officers were satisfied. My *manner* had convinced them. I was singularly at ease. They sat, and while I answered cheerily, they chatted of familiar things. But, ere long, I felt myself getting pale and wished them gone. My head ached, and I fancied a ringing in my ears: but still they sat and still chatted. The ringing became more distinct: I talked more freely to get rid of the feeling: but it continued and gained definitiveness—until, at length, I found that the noise was *not* within my ears.

No doubt I now grew *very* pale;—but I talked more fluently, and with a heightened voice. Yet the sound increased—and what could I do? It was *a low, dull, quick sound—much such a sound as a watch makes when enveloped in cotton.* I gasped for breath—and yet the officers heard it not. I talked more quickly—more vehemently; but the noise steadily increased. I arose and argued about trifles, in a high key and with violent gesticulations; but the noise steadily increased. Why *would* they not be gone? I paced the floor to and fro with heavy strides, as if excited to fury by the observations of the men—but the noise steadily increased. Oh God! what *could* I do? I foamed—I raved—I swore! I swung the chair upon which I had sat, and grated it upon the boards, but the noise arose over all and continually increased. It grew louder—louder—*louder!* And still the men chatted pleasantly, and smiled. Was it possible they heard not? Almighty God!—no, no! They heard!—they suspected!—they *knew!*—they were making a mockery of my horror!—this I thought, and this I think. But anything better than this agony! Anything was more tolerable than this derision! I could bear those hypocritical smiles no longer! I felt that I must scream or die!—and now—again! —hark! louder! louder! louder! *louder!*—

"Villains!" I shrieked, "dissemble no more! I admit the deed!—tear up the planks!—here, here!—it is the beating of his hideous heart!"

The heart of a fool is in his mouth, but the mouth of the wise man is in his heart.
–Benjamin Franklin

THE PUREST THEATRE

Of all the body's organs, writes surgeon Richard Selzer, "the heart is purest theatre, one is quick to concede, throbbing in its cage palpably as any nightingale. It quickens in response to the emotions. Let danger threaten, and the thrilling heart skips a beat or two and tightrope-walks arhythmically before lurching back into the forceful thump of fight or flight. And all the while we feel it, hear it even—we, its stage and its audience."

THE GARRULOUS HEART

by Richard Selzer, M.D.

". . . Across the diaphragm and into the chest . . . here at last is all noise; the whisper of the lungs, the lubdup, lubdup *of the garrulous heart.*

"But it is good you do not hear the machinery of your marrow lest it madden like the buzzing of a thousand coppery bees. It is frightening to lie with your ear in the pillow, and hear the beating of your heart. Not that it beats . . . but that it might stop, even as you listen. For anything that moves must come to rest; no rhythm is endless but must one day lurch . . . then halt. Not that it is a disservice to a man to be made mindful of his death, but—at three o'clock in the morning it is less than philosophy. It is Fantasy, replete with dreadful images forming in the smoke of alabaster crematoria. It is then that one thinks of the bristlecone pines, and envies them for having lasted. It is their slowness, I think. Slow down, heart, and drub on."

Sounds the Heart Makes

Art is long, and Time is fleeting,
And our hearts, though stout and brave,
Still, like muffled drums, are beating
Funeral marches to the grave.
—Henry Wadsworth Longfellow

Few sounds are as familiar to us as that of the heartbeat. It is one of the first (perhaps *the* first) sounds we hear, and throughout life it remains readily identifiable. But what exactly is it? The "lubb dubb" sound of the heart comes from vibrations passing outward from the heart into the chest wall. The first heart sound ("lubb") is produced by the backflow of blood in the ventricles when the ventricular valves close. As the valves close, blood that has been surging forward is suddenly driven back. This sets up a vibration in the walls of the ventricles, and the vibration travels outward, passing into the chest wall where it is attached to the heart. The vibration in the chest wall creates sound waves which, when monitored with the aid of a stethoscope, sound like "lubb."

The second heart sound ("dubb") is created by the vibrations caused by the forceful reverberation of the blood between the arterial walls and the heart valves when the pulmonic and aortic semilunar valves shut. These vibrations, different in tenor from the vibrations set up in the ventricles, pass into the chest wall, are transformed into sound waves, and come out sounding like "dubb."

The "dubb" follows "lubb" after only a brief pause. But a pause twice as long occurs between "dubb" and the next "lubb." During the pause the valves are open, and the blood that passes through them is silent to our ears.

The Walking Heart

A study by Dr. Ralph S. Paffenberger of Stanford University School of Medicine indicates that strenuous exercises decrease the chances of heart attack. The following activities, in increasing value of heart attack prevention, are indicated:

1. Strolling at 1 m.p.h. and walking at 2 m.p.h.
2. Golf, using a power cart.
3. Cleaning windows, mopping floors, and vacuuming.
4. Bowling.
5. Walking at 3 m.p.h. and cycling at 6 m.p.h.
6. Golf, using a pull-cart.
7. Scrubbing floors.
8. Walking at 3.5 m.p.h. and cycling at 8 m.p.h.
9. Golf, carrying clubs.
10. Tennis doubles.
11. Walking at 4 m.p.h., cycling at 10 m.p.h., and ice or roller skating.
12. Walking at 5 m.p.h. and cycling at 11 m.p.h.
13. Tennis singles.
14. Jogging at 5 m.p.h. and cycling at 12 m.p.h.
15. Downhill skiing.
16. Running at 5.5 m.p.h. and cycling at 13 m.p.h.
17. Running at 6 or more m.p.h.
18. Swimming.

"Most of us do not realize that even moderate slopes cause the heart to work harder, helping to raise the pulse rate to what we consider the target or training-effect zone," says Dr. Borisse Paulin. "If the heart is made to beat within this zone for a half-hour or more a day, its stamina increases. In fact, the total cardiovascular system becomes more efficient."

Your "target zone" is easy to compute: It is 70 to 75 percent of your maximum heartbeat. For a twenty-year-old, the maximum heart rate is 200 beats per minute, so the target zone would be 140–150 beats per minute. (The maximum heart rate is 200 beats; for each year after twenty, the maximum decreases approximately one beat per minute.) An exercise or training pulse rate of 70 to 75 percent of your age-related maximum is comfortable and safe for most walkers who are in good health. Unless you are training for the Olympics, exercising vigorously enough to bring your heart rate up to near-maximum is unnecessary, and for most people impossible. It is a good idea to check with your doctor before beginning any vigorous exercise program.

As the arteries grow hard, the heart grows soft. –H.L. Mencken

Heart-to-Heart

In 1968, Myron Brenton published a book entitled *Sex and Your Heart* in which he cited some very interesting research. One study, conducted by Boas and Goldschmidt, measured the heart rate of a couple engaged in sex and concluded what many people had already suspected—that intercourse can be one of the most strenuous activities around.

The average resting heart rate is about 70 beats per minute, but when the subjects of the study began their sexual activity their heart rates were already at 90, and these rates reached higher levels with each orgasm, eventually climbing to almost 150. Certainly more taxing than a cold shower, which averages a maximum heart rate of somewhere around 105!

Great thoughts come from the heart.

–Luc de Clapiers, Marquis de Vauvenargues

Some people feel with their heads and think with their hearts.

–G.C. Lichtenberg

The hearts of holy men are temples in the truth of things, and, in type and shadow, they are heaven itself.

–Jeremy Taylor

A noble heart, like the sun, showeth its greatest countenance in its lowest estate.

–Sir Philip Sidney

The Healthy Heart

Heart attack is a non-specific term that usually refers to a myocardial infarction.

One out of every four heart attack deaths strikes someone under the age of 65; one out of every six stroke victims is under the age of 65.

Heart disease and its widespread effects cost the country about 28 billion dollars a year.

Of the 24 million Americans suffering from high blood pressure, at least 7 million are not even aware that they have the problem.

No heart attack is ever really "sudden." It may seem that way to the patient and family members, but coronary disease has in all likelihood been building over the years, helped along by the patient who has ignored the risk factors and failed to heed the early warning signals.
–American Heart Association

KNOW THE WARNING SIGNALS OF A HEART ATTACK

—Uncomfortable pressure, fullness, squeezing or pain in the center of your chest, lasting two minutes or more.

—Pain may spread to shoulders, neck or arms.

—Severe pain, dizziness, fainting, sweating, nausea, or shortness of breath may also occur.

Not all these signals, however, are always present. **Don't wait.** *Get help immediately. Information courtesy of the American Heart Association.*

BE A HEART SAVER

You'll want to take immediate action if you or one of your loved ones feels the warning signals of a heart attack (see p. 90). The American Heart Association (National Center, 7320 Greenville Avenue, Dallas Texas 75231) offers these guidelines:

—If you are with someone who is having the "signals," and if they last for two minutes or longer, act at once.

—Expect a "denial." It is normal to deny the possibility of anything as serious as a heart attack—but insist on taking prompt action.

—Call the emergency rescue service, or

—Get to the nearest hospital emergency room that offers 24-hour emergency cardiac care.

—Give mouth-to-mouth breathing and chest compression (CPR) if it is necessary and if you are properly trained.

BE PREPARED

—Find out which hospitals in your area offer 24-hour emergency cardiac care.

—Select in advance the facility nearest your home and office and tell your family and friends so that they will know what to do.

—Keep a list of emergency rescue service numbers next to your telephone and in a prominent place in your pocket, wallet or purse.

—Learn CPR.

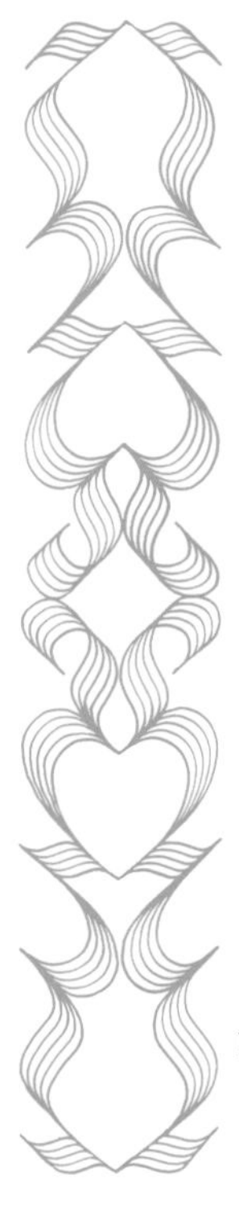

BROADWAY HEARTS

Can you select the musical show in which each of the following heart songs appears?

1. "A Dream Is a Wish Your Heart Makes." (a) *Frankie and Johnny,* (b) *A Tree Grows in Brooklyn,* (c) *Disneyland,* (d) *The Fantasticks.*
2. "Heart (You Gotta Have Heart)." (a) *Can-Can,* (b) *Plain and Fancy,* (c) *Seventeen,* (d) *Damn Yankees.*
3. "My Heart Belongs to Daddy." (a) *Leave It to Me,* (b) *Fiddler on the Roof,* (c) *Sweethearts,* (d) *L'il Abner.*
4. "My Heart Is Full of You." (a) *All For Love,* (b) *Most Happy Fella,* (c) *Fanny,* (d) *Always in My Heart.*
5. "My Heart Stood Still." (a) *Connecticut Yankees,* (b) *Oklahoma,* (c) *Three Coins in the Fountain,* (d) *You're a Sweetheart.*
6. "Raining in My Heart." (a) *My Fair Lady,* (b) *Carefree Heart,* (c) *The Student Prince,* (d) *Dames at Sea.*
7. "Two Hearts Are Better Than One." (a) *Merry Widow,* (b) *Centennial Summer,* (c) *South Pacific,* (d) *The World of Charles Aznavour.*
8. "Way to a Man's Heart." (a) *L'il Abner,* (b) *Carnival,* (c) *One Hour With You,* (d) *High Society.*
9. "With a Song in My Heart." (a) *The Blossom,* (b) *Seventeen,* (c) *Spring Is Here,* (d) *Carefree Heart.*
10. "Zing! Went the Strings of My Heart." (a) *Conversation Piece,* (b) *How To Succeed in Business Without Really Trying,* (c) *Queen High,* (d) *Thumbs Up.*

Answers: 1–c, 2–d, 3–a, 4–b, 5–a, 6–d, 7–b, 8–a, 9–c, 10–d.

Other Hearty Song Titles

"A Headache and a Heart"
"Always in My Heart"
"Can't You Hear My Heart Beat?"
"Cross Your Heart"
"Deep in the Heart of Texas"
"Devil in Her Heart"
"Down in My Heart"
"Drums in My Heart"
"Expressway to Your Heart"
"Follow Your Heart"
"Foolish Heart"
"Give Me a Heart to Sing To"
"Heart and Soul"
"Heart Full of Soul"
"Heartless"
"Heart Like a Wheel"
"Her Heart Was in Her Work"
"Hungry Heart"
"I Let a Song Go Out of My Heart"
"If You Haven't Got a Sweetheart"
"I'll Follow My Secret Heart"
"I've a Strange New Rhythm in My Heart"
"Let Me Call You Sweetheart"
"Little More Heart"
"Love from a Heart of Gold"
"May Your Heart Stay Young"
"My Heart Cries for You"
"My Heart Is Full of You"
"My Heart Is Like a Violin"
"My Heart Leaps Up"
"My Heart Won't Say Goodbye"
"My Heart's a Darlin' "
"My Heart's in the Middle of July"
"Only Love Can Break Your Heart"
"Piece of My Heart"
"Restless Heart"
"Search Your Heart"
"Way to a Man's Heart"
"We Will Always Be Sweethearts"
"When Hearts Are Young"
"Wooden Heart"
"Yes My Heart"
"You Belong to My Heart"
"You Set My Heart to Music"
"You're Breaking My Heart"

First in The Hearts

It was the *Resolutions Presented to the House of Representatives* upon the death of George Washington that carried Henry Lee's famous dedication, "To the memory of the Man, first in war, first in peace, and first in the hearts of his countrymen."

National Observances

§169b. American Heart Month

The President of the United States is authorized and requested to issue annually a proclamation (1) designating February as American Heart Month, (2) inviting the Governors of the States and territories of the United States to issue proclamations for like purposes, and (3) urging the people of the United States to give heed to the nationwide problem of the heart and blood vessel diseases, and to support all essential programs required to bring about its solution.

CROSS MY HEART

ACROSS

1 *Catch sight of*
5 *"Act One" author*
10 *Gives courage to*
14 *Gambler, in old Rome*
15 *Miss Loos*
16 *Victim*
17 *N.Z. bird*
18 *French historian*
19 *Kilns*
20 *Pitiable*
22 *Most arid*
24 *Spur*
25 *"Unto us ______ is given"*
26 *Coneys*
29 *Dauntless*
33 *Gladden*
34 *Walk pompously*
35 *Busy one*
36 *Extremely generous*
37 *Trompe ______; visual deception*
38 *Roll up, as a flag*
39 *Type of novel: Abbr.*
40 *Burmese rices*
41 *Mr. Puzo*
42 *Frank discussion*
44 *French queens*
45 *Adriatic wind*
46 *Writer O'Casey*
47 *Iran's capital*
50 *Carefree*
54 *French thought*
55 *Cape Verde island*
57 *"The ______ Lonely Hunter"*
58 *Concert halls*
59 *City of China*
60 *Otherwise*
61 *Polio pioneer*
62 *Unfeeling*
63 *Colorist*

DOWN

1 *Flier Amelia*
2 *Cast aspersions on*
3 ______ *Marquette*

(Answer to puzzle will be found on page 18.)

4 *Lively in spite of age*
5 *Miss Tallchief* et al.
6 *Upright*
7 *"Wake Up and ________"*
8 *Depot: Abbr.*
9 *Completely*
10 *Center of an escutcheon*
11 *Gaelic*
12 *Butterfly and hair*
13 *Part of C.B.S.: Abbr.*
21 *Finished*
23 *Defeat soundly*
25 *Prefixes for heart cavities*
26 *Words of affection*
27 *Apportion*
28 *Swedish port*
29 *Salisbury________*
30 *Aftermath of overeating*
31 *Uncanny*
32 *Apollo's birthplace*
34 *Fa follower*
37 *Memorize*
38 *Timorous*
40 *Portico*
41 *Biblical wall tower*
43 *Sorrow*
44 *Lear's daughter* et al.
46 *Hindu deity and others*
47 *Spanish uncles*
48 *Icelandic writing*
49 *Cad*
50 *Superman's Lois*
51 *Cordially*
52 *Common Latin verb*
53 *Of stock, in old Ireland*
56 *Aunt or uncle: Abbr.*

HEARTS OF GOLD

(Based on a Million Sales)

Year	Song	Artist
1956	"Heartbreak Hotel"	Elvis Presley
1957	"That's When Your Heartache Begins"	Elvis Presley
1963	"I Left My Heart in San Francisco"	Tony Bennett
1965	"Dear Heart"	Andy Williams
1967	"Sergeant Pepper's Lonely Hearts Club Band"	The Beatles
1969	"Your Cheatin' Heart"	Hank Williams
"	"Put a Little Love in Your Heart"	Jackie DeShannon
"	"Happy Heart"	Andy Williams
1971	"Sweetheart"	Englebert Humperdinck
"	"How Can You Mend A Broken Heart?"	The Bee Gees
1972	"Charley Pride Sings Heart Songs"	Charley Pride
"	"Heart of Gold"	Neil Young
1973	"Heartbeat—It's a Lovebeat"	The DeFranco Family
1975	"Sheer Heart Attack"	Queen
1976	"Don't Go Breaking My Heart"	Elton John & Kiki Dee
1978	"You're in My Heart"	Rod Stewart
"	"It's a Heartache"	Bonnie Tyler
1979	"Heart of Glass"	Blondie
1981	"Heartache Tonight"	Eagles
1982	"Queen of Hearts"	Juice Newton

WITH A HEART IN MY SONG

Match the following heart songs with the recording artists who made them popular.

SONG	ARTIST
1. "Cold, Cold Heart"	a. Rolling Stones
2. "Crazy Heart"	b. Mary Martin
3. "Heart of My Heart"	c. Barbra Streisand
4. "Heart of Stone"	d. Hank Williams
5. "Heart on the Line"	e. Peter Frampton
6. "My Heart Belongs to Daddy"	f. Hill & Range
7. "My Heart Belongs to Me"	g. Frank Sinatra
8. "Peg O' My Heart"	h. Hank Williams
9. "This Heart of Mine"	i. Four Aces
10. "Young at Heart"	j. Leo Fesit

ANSWERS: 1-d, 2-h, 3-i, 4-a, 5-e, 6-b, 7-c, 8-j, 9-f, 10-g.